How Healers Heal

Lifestyle Medicine Physicians Transforming
Healthcare and Their Own Health

Compiled and Edited by

Shilpi Pradhan, MD

The front cover design was done by Dr. Cherie Chu.

The back cover design was done by Dr. Shilpi Pradhan.

E-book ISBN: 978-1-961549-00-5

Paperback ISBN: 978-1-961549-01-2

Hardback ISBN: 978-1-961549-02-9

This book is written with the collective goal of the authors to be a fundraiser. Profits from the first year of sales will be donated to the American College of Lifestyle Medicine (ACLM) up to $10,000.

All websites were accurate at the time of publication of this book. Any changes in the future cannot be accounted for at the time of publication. Hyperlinks on the ebook version to other books on Amazon may be Amazon Affiliate links.

The authors would like to dedicate this book to their patients, who are instrumental in their learning and inspire them daily.

And to their spouses, partners, families, friends, coworkers, and everyone who made their journeys possible.

Co-Authors

Qadira Malika Ali, MD, MPH, DipABLM

Shruthi Chandrashekhar, MD, DipABOM, DipABLM

Cherie Chu, MD, FAAP, DipABLM

Nupur Garg, MD, DipABLM

Prachi Garodia, MD, ABIM, ABIHM, DipABLM, DipAyu, NBC-HWC

Sirisha Guthikonda, MD, DipABLM

Kelley Hagerich, MD, MPH, FACP, DipABOM, DipABLM

Teresa Hardisty, MD, FAAP, DipABLM

Claudine Holt, MD, MPH, DipABLM

Julia Huber, MD, DipABLM, TIPC

Geetha Kamath, MD, FACP, DipABLM, DipABOM

Mitika Kanabar MD, MPH, FASAM, DipABLM

Mary Anne Kiel, MD, FAAP, DipABLM, CPE

Simran Malhotra, MD, DipABLM, CHWC

Erin Mayfield, DO, DipABLM, DipAOBOG

Khyati Mehta, MD, DipABLM

Anjali Nakra, MBBS, DO, DipIBLM

Lisa Pathak, MD, FACP, FAAP, DipABLM

Amy Patel, MD, FAAP, DipABIM, DipABLM

Karmi Patel, MD, FACP, DipABLM

Gouri Pimputkar, DO, FACOOG, DipABLM

Shilpi Pradhan, MD, DipABLM

Supriya Rao, MD, DipABLM, DipABOM

Tatyana Reznik, MD, FACP, DipABLM

Trisha Schimek, MD, MSPH, DipABLM

Wendy Schofer, MD, FAAP, DipABLM, TIPC, CHWC

Mythri Shankar, MD, DipIBLM, AFMCP

Saba Sharif, MD, FAAAI, DipABLM

Mamatha Sirivol, MD, MPH, DipABLM, DipABOM

Wendy Stammers (UK), MBCHB, MRCGP, DFSRH, DRCOG, Dip-IBLM/BSLM

Nandini Sunkireddy, MD, DipABLM, DipABOM

Yolandas Renee Thomason, DO, DipABOM, DipABLM

Jaya Venkataraman, MD, FAAP, DipABLM

Preface

Did you know the adult obesity rate is 41.9% and the child obesity rate is 19.7% in the United States, according to the Centers for Disease Control (CDC)? Did you know that obesity-related diseases can be reversible and treatable without medications? Did you know that healthcare professionals (HCP) are more likely to experience burnout than any other profession, according to the CDC? Have you heard of Lifestyle Medicine and how it can be a solution for burnout? Do you wonder how people turn their lives around and how you can do the same?

Then keep reading . . .

In this book, you'll discover:

- Six pillars of health and tips on how to achieve them.

- An evidence-based approach to everything your mother told you to do.

- Stories of struggle and positivity in overcoming health challenges.

- How Lifestyle Medicine (LM) can be the cure for HCP burnout.

- How LM board certification can help healthcare professionals change their lives and the lives of patients.

- And much more!

This book, *How Healers Heal*, was a project conceived by Dr. Pradhan and Dr. Sharif in January 2023 about how transformative Lifestyle Medicine has been in our lives, and with shared enthusiasm from Dr. Huber and Dr. Sunkireddy, this book project was born.

In this book, you'll read deeply personal stories from 33 board-certified Lifestyle Medicine physicians about how they are changing their lives and the lives of their patients using the six pillars of health with Lifestyle Medicine. You'll discover narratives about these physicians' life-changing events like chest pain, infertility, loss of loved ones, COVID, immune deficiency, alopecia, burnout, and much more, along with how the events were catalysts for their health transformations.

Rising rates of obesity and their related metabolic illnesses of diabetes, hypertension, stroke, dementia, and autoimmune disease are on the rise in the United States right when physician burnout is at an all-time record high. Lifestyle Medicine could be the perfect catalyst for change in a failing healthcare system. A movement of physicians is bringing back the focus to lifestyle medicine and prevention, and it has already proven to improve the lives of these physicians and their countless patients.

If you're ready to be inspired, then grab a seat and keep reading!

Check out our website for interviews with the authors!

www.HowHealersHeal.com

CONTENTS

PRAISE FOR HOW HEALERS HEAL

———◆◇◆———

"It warms my heart to read stories of women physicians using my life's work, especially harnessing the power of nutrition provided by the whole food plant-based diet, to ground the wholistic perspectives on human health to serve their families, their communities and themselves." — Dr. T. Colin Campbell, Ph.D., Jacob Gould Schurman Professor, Emeritus of Nutritional Biochemistry, Cornell University, Author of Forks Over Knives: The Plant-Based Way to Health, The China Study, The Low-Carb Fraud, Whole: Rethinking the Science of Nutrition and many other books.

———◆◇◆———

"This inspiring book shares the personal and professional passion of healthcare professionals choosing to care for themselves and their patients in a more holistic way. The true healing power of healthy lifestyle habits is laid bare, leaving no doubt that both physical and mental well-being can be achieved through the practice of lifestyle medicine. A must-read for clinicians and patients who will find themselves motivated to make powerful changes to their own lifestyles and support others to do the same." — Dr. Shireen Kassam, MBBS, PhD, FRCPath, DipIBLM, Haematologist and

Lifestyle Medicine Physician, Author of <u>Eating Plant-Based</u>.

———◆◇◆———

"These amazing authors have shared their stories about how lifestyle medicine impacted their lives and helped them renew their sense of purpose, in some cases escaping burnout and in all cases becoming passionate about the six pillars of lifestyle medicine. Reading about each author's unique journey with lifestyle medicine is inspirational!" — <u>Dr. Beth Frates</u>, MD, DipABLM, President of the American College of Lifestyle Medicine (2022-2024), Author of <u>The Lifestyle Medicine Handbook</u>, and many other books.

———◆◇◆———

"This remarkable book offers inspiring stories of 33 courageous women physicians who have transformed their personal and professional lives by integrating lifestyle medicine. Their honesty, resilience, and vulnerability are captivating. Each chapter beautifully weaves challenges, triumphs, and moments of self-discovery. It is not just a compilation of stories but a call to action for all physicians to prioritize their well-being and integrate lifestyle medicine into patient care. It rekindles our passion for medicine and empowers us to guide our patients toward healthier and more fulfilling lives." — Dr. Padmaja Patel, MD, FACLM, DipABLM, Lifestyle Medicine Medical Director, <u>Wellvana</u>; President-Elect (2024-2026), American College of Lifestyle Medicine; Vice President, World Lifestyle Medicine Organization; Certified Lifestyle Medicine Intensivist.

———◆◇◆———

"Self-care through lifestyle medicine lights the way for clinicians, women and men alike, to navigate both the demands and immense joys of their professional and personal lives. These women share sometimes powerful, sometimes tender, and always deeply personal stories on their paths to healing and regaining hope in their lives. Every clinician will see themselves in one or many of the journeys shared, and all will find uplifting inspiration in these pages." — Dr. Catherine Collings, MD, FACC, MS, DipABLM; Chief Medical Officer, HealthFleet; Immediate Past President (2020-2022) and Board of Directors, <u>American College of Lifestyle Medicine</u>.

———————◆○◆———————

"This distinctive series of unforgettable health transformation stories is truly a gift! The authors' sincerity and vulnerability in sharing their challenges about their health, their professions, and their personal lives, and the significant successes they achieved through Lifestyle Medicine, is especially moving. I can identify with and appreciate these bold women physicians, given my own personal journey and triumphs with whole food plant-based eating. I believe this book will be a great resource for others (both healthcare professionals and patients) who are searching for solutions to similar challenges." — Gwyn Whittaker, CEO, <u>GreenFare Organic Café</u> and Executive Producer, The Game Changers and Eating Our Way to Extinction.

———————◆○◆———————

"The stories these authors candidly share is a testament to the true healing power of lifestyle medicine personally and professionally. Their journeys are inspiring and a call to action for integrating the pillars into our lives and work. It's life-changing recommended reading!" — Dr. Sharon Horesh Bergquist, MD, Pam R. Rollins Professor of Medicine at Emory

University and co-author of <u>Plantology: A cookbook based on the science of plant-based eating</u>.

———◆———

"I'm delighted that this collection of truly transformational stories by women lifestyle medicine physicians is here to emphasize the critical need of our health care community to restore our own health, in addition to that of our patients. Their focus on the six pillars of lifestyle medicine, but especially the pillar of nutrition through whole food plant predominant eating, sends a powerful message about how we can restore and maintain our vitality, longevity, and passion for medicine." — Dr. James F. Loomis, MD, MBA, DipABLM, FACLM, Medical Director, Barnard Medical Center, Washington, DC.

———◆———

"This book has deeply moved me. The personal accounts it contains are more than just stories - they are profound journeys of transformation through lifestyle medicine. Each physician's tale is a testament to resilience, a narrative of facing health challenges head-on and emerging not just healed, but renewed. These stories are raw, real, and deeply inspiring. They remind us that we are not just practitioners, but healers, and, at times, patients. This book is also a glimpse into the future of medicine. In the telling of these stories, we see the birth of an evolved healthcare system, one that empowers individuals to take control of their health and find joy in the journey. This book is a heartfelt exploration of that potential. If you're seeking a book that will move you, challenge you, and change your perspective on health, this is it. It's a compelling glimpse into the future of medicine, and I can't recommend it enough." — Dr. Rakesh (Dr. Rak ("rock")) Jotwani, MD, DipABLM. Host of <u>The Healthy Feast podcast</u>, former Director of Lifestyle Medicine at Kaiser Permanente San

Francisco

"Finally, a book that demonstrates the power of lifestyle medicine... not just for our patients but for ourselves as well. Combined with the strength and energy of the collaboration of women physicians, this book is bound to be a tipping point in health care and physician wholeness. What lifestyle medicine reveals is the opportunity to get back to the roots of dis-ease and to refocus on the building blocks of physician and emotional health - whole foods as fuel, consistent movement, restorative sleep, mindful stress reduction, avoidance of toxic substances, and social connectedness. We envision a future of strong, rejuvenated physicians able to help our patients achieve the same. This book is a spotlight onto that reality to come." — Dr. Heather Hammerstedt MD, MPH, FACEP, DipABLM, Emergency Medicine/ Lifestyle Medicine/ Integrative Nutrition Coach, CEO Wholist

---

"This book is a gift! These are real stories of doctors who are changing their lives, the lives of the patients, and now whole communities. This is a book to not only buy a copy of but gift copies to the people in your life." — Dr. Nneka Unachukwu, MD, Founder, EntreMD Business School; CEO, Ivy League Pediatrics; Author, The EntreMD Method and Made for More.

"You will find medicine at a precipice these days between medications and wellness battling in all socioeconomic classes. These doctors and these stories are so personal and powerful that you will find yourself leaning into your

power and true choice to find your own path to wellness and true health. And these stories show Lifestyle Medicine as a path out of burnout as well. A must read" — Dr. Sharon McLaughlin, MD, Founder of Female Physician Entrepreneurs; Author/compiler of the book Thriving after Burnout.

<hr>

"This is a book about hope. Inspiring stories from physicians who have changed their own lives with lifestyle medicine and are changing the face of medicine to be a whole-body approach that encompasses nutrition, genetics, social connection, and much more into a patient's care. From learning to cook for their families, googling their symptoms, to creating daily healthy habits that will transcend generations, these amazing stories will inspire you to redefine health for you, your family, and your patients." — Dr. Jennifer Roelands, MD, SHEO of Well Woman MD, direct integrative medicine practice, podcast host *Ignite Your Powher*, and go-to math guru to 4 amazing kids.

<hr>

"In the current state of healthcare, it has never been more important and urgent that we take care of our physicians and healthcare team. This compilation of physicians who have lived the full life experiences brings to our attention the humanism of our healthcare professionals and what each of them has done first to heal themselves AND now to empower us all to do the same. Thank you for doing this for all of us." — Dr. Latifat Akintade, MD, Founder of MoneyFitMD; Author, Done with Broke: The Woman Physician's Guide to More Money and Less Hustle.

———◆O◆———

"So much of our future rests on our adherence to principles of healthy living that can prevent and reverse disease. These inspiring physicians have educated themselves on what they did not receive in their training, and they are now blessing their patients with this knowledge. Their stories, quotes, and valuable resources will transform your life if you choose to act on what is available through this book!" — Dr. Ann Huntington, MD, FACP, is an internist and lifestyle and integrative medicine enthusiast. She is the Founder of Give More Naturally (www.givemorenaturally.com) and the co-author of the book Thriving After Burnout.

———◆O◆———

"At a time when our healthcare system is experiencing crisis levels of health worker burnout, How Healers Heal offers a window into the power of Lifestyle Medicine. Evidence-based, proven, and remarkably simple, the principles of Lifestyle Medicine make so much sense, not only for the well-being and health of our patients but also for the well-being and longevity of our healers. Through personal, engaging, and vulnerable stories, the physicians in this book share their own journeys to finding, sharing, and embodying Lifestyle Medicine in all its potential. I wish I had discovered Lifestyle Medicine years ago, and am grateful to the authors for spreading the word so that we all can learn, heal and create a brighter future together." — Dr. Tammie Chang, MD, Co-Founder Pink Coat, MD; Medical Director, MultiCare Physician/APP Wellness; Author, Boundaries for Women Physicians; Speaker, Coach, Pediatric Hematologist/Oncologist.

———◄◦►———

"The stories these authors candidly share is a testament to the true healing power of lifestyle medicine personally and professionally. Their journeys are inspiring and a call to action for integrating the pillars into our lives and work. It's life-changing recommended reading!" — Dr. Sharon Horesh Bergquist, MD, Pam R. Rollins Professor of Medicine at Emory University and co-author of Plantology: A cookbook based on the science of plant-based eating.

———◄◦►———

"This is a beautiful contribution, and I'm sure it will help many. I got on this topic and journey myself after witnessing how my mother suffered with "medical treatment" that were supposedly comfort approach but yet not! My years of medical training, experience, and triple board certifications seem limited! Current medical care has not been nourishing for the spirits & soul at all and minimally touching the physical aspect too. I think Lifestyle Medicine is a remarkable breakthrough and surely the way for healthcare in the current and future times to come. Wish you and all the co-authors very much success. Thanks for sharing this valuable knowledge with me!" — Dr. Aparna Ranjan, MD, Geriatric Medicine, Hospice and Palliative Care, and Internal Medicine Doctor.

———◄◦►———

Introduction

"With knowledge comes power, and with power comes great responsibility."

— Adage from many civilizations

Thank you for choosing to read our stories of transformation. These stories are full of hope and have made the difference between life and death for some of us. All of these transformations have occurred because of Lifestyle Medicine. Lifestyle Medicine is a relatively new field in medicine; however, it collects everything we already know about what we should be doing and what our moms have told us, like eating more vegetables, and applies evidence-based medicine to those ideas and proves them worthy. This book explores the six pillars of Lifestyle Medicine with a personal touch as we share our stories of transformation using a scientifically backed approach to health and well-being that emphasizes the role of lifestyle in the prevention, treatment, and reversal of chronic diseases.

"The American College of Lifestyle Medicine (ACLM) is the medical professional society for physicians and other professionals dedicated to clinical and worksite practice of lifestyle medicine as the foundation of a transformed and sustainable healthcare system" (www.lifestylemedicine.org). All the co-authors you will read about in this book are board-certified in the field of Lifestyle Medicine either by the American Board of Lifestyle Medicine or the International Board of Lifestyle Medicine, in addition to their primary specialty in various fields of medicine.

Six pillars of health that anchor Lifestyle Medicine are:

1. Nutrition,

2. Physical Activity,

3. Stress Management,

4. Restorative Sleep,

5. Social Connections, and

6. Avoidance of Risky Substances.

NUTRITION

"When diet is wrong, medicine is of no use. When diet is correct, medicine is of no need."

— Ayurvedic Proverb

Nutrition is the foundation of good health. One surprising fact we've learned is that lifestyle changes can actually reverse disease. Our bodies are so powerful that if we give them the proper nutrients, they can actually heal themselves. This is different from what we learned in medical school about chronic diseases as progressive and irreversible. The recommended diet is predominantly a whole food and plant-based (WFPB) diet for humans. This means eating food that is in its least processed state, like a whole apple instead of applesauce or apple juice. A nutritionally-rich diet helps you improve your heart health, manage your weight better, improve your cognitive function (yes, the nutrients in whole food help you think better and can prevent dementia), reduce your risk of chronic diseases like diabetes, and improve your gut health for a better microbiome which nourishes you from the inside.

A stark contrast to this is the Standard American Diet (SAD) that most Americans are accustomed to consuming. Fortunately, this is rapidly changing with education, like in this book, and the numerous resources from the leaders of the Lifestyle Medicine movement. The SAD is characterized by high amounts of processed and refined foods, sugar, and unhealthy fats. The SAD raises cholesterol levels and the risk of heart attacks, and contributes to insulin resistance which then leads to metabolic syndrome and possibly type 2 diabetes. The SAD is a major factor in the obesity epidemic. According to the Centers for Disease Control (CDC), the rate of obesity among American adults is estimated to be 41.9%, while among children the obesity rate is 19.7% and growing. This means 2 out of every 5 Americans would be considered obese. Those are staggering numbers, and they will keep growing if we don't take back our health. The SAD also elevates blood pressure which can lead to stroke and chronic kidney disease. The SAD lacks dietary fiber, which protects against colon cancer and helps your gut microbiome. The SAD also has highly carcinogenic food like charred and processed meat, which can increase the risk of cancer, specifically colon cancer. The World Health Organization (WHO) has classified processed meat as a carcinogen. We need to ask ourselves — why is it still sold in grocery stores and deli chains?

In contrast, adopting a whole food, plant-based diet (WFPBD) not only has numerous benefits for our personal health and well-being, but it also has a positive impact on the environment and future generations. A plant-based diet requires fewer resources and produces fewer greenhouse gas emissions than a diet heavy on animal products, thus helping reduce our impact on climate change. In addition, plant-based diets promote sustainable agriculture and reduce the use of harmful pesticides and fertilizers, which in turn helps protect soil and water quality. By eating a diet rich in whole, plant-based foods, we can help create a more sustainable and healthier future for ourselves and the planet.

While food can, at times, be a polarizing topic, being healthy should not be controversial. While not all of the authors in this book have adopted a completely vegan diet, we have made bold food choices for our own health and those we care about. We strongly prefer and recommend WFPB diets or "plant-predominant" or "plant-forward" diets. We feel a sense of duty to educate about the positive impact our food choices can have on our health. We are here to help you discover a new path, giving you the information to make the best choice for your life and health. As Jackie Robinson says, "Life is not a spectator sport. If you're going to spend your whole life in the grandstand watching what goes on, in my opinion, you're wasting your life." We are ready to help you with our stories and lead by example.

PHYSICAL ACTIVITY

"If you don't make time for exercise, you'll probably have to make time for illness."

— Robin Sharma

The role of exercise in improving health and preventing chronic diseases is well known. The recommended 150 minutes of moderate physical activity per week is supported by Lifestyle Medicine. What does moderate exercise mean? It means while doing that activity, you get slightly out of breath, as you cannot sing but can still talk. Ideally, we split up the 150 minutes into five 30-minute increments and not one long session once a week.

We know when we move our bodies, the effects are palpable right away in how we feel. Aerobic exercise releases endorphins and other hormones, which actually lower blood pressure, lower your cholesterol level, and therefore reduce your risk of heart disease and stroke. We can feel those endorphins improve our mood. They also trigger feelings of happiness which can help reduce our overall stress, anxiety, and depression. Did you know exercise can also improve how your brain actually functions and your long-term memory?

We also know stretching exercises and various forms of yoga help build our muscles and improve flexibility. It is recommended to stretch all major muscle groups for 10 minutes each, two to three times per week, and hold the stretch for 10-30 seconds, repeating each muscle group two to three times. For healthy adults, the recommended strength training is 2-3 times per week on non-consecutive days for 8-12 repetitions of all major muscle groups. Major muscle groups include the chest, back, shoulders, biceps, triceps, abdomen, quadriceps, and hamstrings. Think of exercise as a medication you have prescribed for yourself.

Stronger muscles help improve the stability of our joints. This, in turn, helps decrease the long-term risk of joint injury. Exercise also helps us burn fat and manage our goal of maintaining a healthy weight. By maintaining a healthy weight, we can reduce the risk of obesity and its associated diseases like diabetes. Exercise can also help improve our immune system and help us overcome viral and bacterial infections quicker.

Regular physical activity serves as a bridge for establishing social connections. When we exercise with our friends, like training for and running a 5K race or playing pickleball, we build valuable social connections. By incorporating regular physical activity into our lives, we can reap numerous physical, social, and mental health benefits and improve our overall quality of life. Exercise brings balance to our bodies and optimizes our bodies. It's as easy as going out for a walk. So, let's go move our bodies!

STRESS MANAGEMENT

"Do something today that your future self will thank you for."

— Sean Patrick Flanery

Stress is an inevitable part and parcel of daily life, but how we manage it can have a significant impact on our health and well-being. Undue and poorly managed stress can have devastating consequences for our home and professional lives. Chronic stress can lead to various negative health outcomes, including an increased risk of heart disease, depression, anxiety, and other mental health conditions. It can also weaken the immune system and increase inflammation in the body. Effective stress management can help reduce these negative impacts and improve overall health and well-being. Lifestyle Medicine recognizes that controlling stress is as important as nutrition and physical exercise for our body and mind. For some of you, this may mean a certain spiritual or religious practice, or perhaps writing a daily journal or even meditation. This and other practices of stress management may be combined with physical exercise to improve the well-being of each individual. All of us have different ways of how we can meet this need, but addressing it on a daily basis is crucial to our overall health.

> "When we practice mindfulness, our thoughts tune in to what we're sensing in the present moment rather than rehashing the past or imagining the future."
> — Brené Brown, Rising Strong

The pillars of LM also intertwine, as we all know about stress eating and eating food that may be unhealthy and sugary, which increases our dopamine and feel-good hormones temporarily, however, may not be good for our bodies in the long term. Managing stress also means finding a healthy coping mechanism rather than eating unhealthy processed foods. As we build healthy habits into our daily routine for stress management, the urge to stress eat will also decrease.

RESTORATIVE SLEEP

"Innocent sleep. Sleep that soothes away all our worries. Sleep that puts each day to rest. Sleep that relieves the weary laborer and heals hurt minds. Sleep, the main course in life's feast, and the most nourishing."
— William Shakespeare, Macbeth

Adequate and quality sleep is essential for good health and optimal daily functioning. The American Academy of Sleep Medicine recommends 7–9 hours of sleep for an average adult (growing children need more sleep). Sleep plays a vital role in our physical and mental recovery and helps restore many functions, including the regeneration of damaged tissues, consolidation of memories, and the processing of emotions and experiences. Your body NEEDS sleep. There's no badge to be earned by sleeping less and doing more, as we may have been taught in our medical training. Your badge should be one of resting and helping your body feel better.

"It's okay to pace yourself, get a little rest, and speak of your struggles out loud. It's ok to prioritize your wellness, to make a habit of rest and repair."
— Michele Obama, The Light We Carry

Lack of sleep or poor sleep quality has been linked to various negative health outcomes, including impaired cognitive function, weakened immune system, increased inflammation, and heightened risk of chronic diseases such as obesity, diabetes, cardiovascular disease, and depression. Yes, not sleeping can increase your body weight. If you're having trouble losing weight, the first pillar of health you need to address may actually be sleep. Sleep deprivation can also lead to mood changes, decreased productivity, and increased risk of accidents and errors at work, while driving a car, and at home. In America, we have become accustomed to working long hours. It is absolutely essential for us to get enough sleep so our bodies can reset and function at their peak level.

SOCIAL CONNECTIONS

> "No man is an island entire of itself; every man is a piece of the continent, a part of the main."
>
> — John Donne

The importance of social connections for mental and physical health may be one of the most important aspects of our overall health, more than nutrition or exercise, in the latest research. This was especially true during the COVID-19 pandemic. Social connectedness refers to the relationships and connections we have with others, including family, friends, and communities. It plays a crucial role in our physical health and mental well-being. Research has shown that strong social connections can reduce stress, improve mood, and increase life satisfaction. Social support also helps people cope with difficult life events and can have a positive impact on physical health. It is also associated with a reduced risk of chronic diseases such as heart disease, stroke, and depression. We can build our social connections while exercising or taking a cooking class, or engaging in a wellness program, unconsciously combining the benefits of many pillars of health into one activity.

On the contrary, social isolation and loneliness have been linked to negative health outcomes such as increased inflammation, poor immune function, and a higher risk of premature death. Especially for healthcare professionals with long work hours, lack of social connection and subsequent isolation can lead to burnout. Maintaining and nurturing a meaningful social network is essential for overall health and well-being, but even a simple smile at a stranger at a grocery store can be uplifting.

Our surgeon general, Dr. Vivek Murthy, has highlighted loneliness as being as deadly as smoking in his recent report, <u>Epidemic of Loneliness and Isolation in the United States</u>, and his book, <u>*Together*</u>. He has laid out a plan for the government to help in a systematic way. This includes policies to 1) "Strengthen Social Infrastructure" like parks and programs, 2) "Enact Pro-Connection Public Policies" like public transportation and paid leave, 3) "Mobilize the Health Sector" by having doctors assess for loneliness, 4) "Reform Digital Environments" by re-evaluating our relationship with technology, 5) "Deepen Our Knowledge" with the research on causes of social disconnection, and 6) "Cultivate a Culture of Connection" by being conscious of our daily interactions.

AVOIDANCE OF RISKY SUBSTANCES

"Nobody stays recovered unless the life they have created is more rewarding and satisfying than the one they left behind."

— Anne Fletcher

The harm caused by tobacco/smoking has been well-known for many decades. Tobacco and other substances prone to possible abuse, such as alcohol and drugs (whether legal or illegal), are also highly addictive. Smoking and the use of harmful substances, such as excessive alcohol and drugs, can negatively impact physical and mental health, increasing the risk of chronic diseases and decreasing our overall quality of life. A detailed discussion of substance abuse and strategies for its mitigation are beyond the scope of this book. Please check out the resources section at the back of the book for many excellent resources to help you quit smoking and deal with other addictions.

PROGRESS

"We are what we repeatedly do. Excellence, then, is not an act, but a habit."

— Aristotle

By embracing these six pillars of health, you will learn how to transform your life, improve your health, and prevent or reverse chronic diseases. Please refer to the section of the book to learn about more resources that can help you on your journey. Feel free to reach out to us individually to learn more, and don't forget to watch videos about our journey to better health. Check out our wellness, coaching, and mentorship program from our experts and take full advantage of their amazing expertise. Feel free to read each author's profile on our website

www.HowHealersHeal.com.

BOARD CERTIFICATION

The field of Lifestyle Medicine is open to all. There are many resources for everyone to learn. If you are a physician, you can become certified by the American Board of Lifestyle Medicine. If you are a health professional with a master's or doctorate in a health or allied health field, you can also become certified by the American College of Lifestyle Medicine. Please check the ACLM website to learn more about certification. If you are a community member, you can help spread messages of hope and health in your community too.

OUR STORIES

In this book, *How Healers Heal*, you will read about how our lives as humans and as physicians have changed using the six pillars of Lifestyle Medicine and how we apply this knowledge to help our families, patients, hospital systems, and the healthcare system at large. We hope to inspire you to take action and change your life and the lives of those around you.

"The best way to predict the future is to create it."
— Abraham Lincoln

We aim to inspire readers to create a healthier, happier future for themselves. Whether that is by adopting a whole food plant-based diet, quitting smoking, strengthening your social connections, or committing to regular exercise. We hope to help you discover that positive change that is within reach for anyone ready to take the first step.

As James Clear says in his book *Atomic Habits*, "If you can get 1 percent better each day for one year, you'll end up thirty-seven times better by the time you're done." Let's keep taking action to help ourselves and our families, one small step at a time.

Sincerely,

Shilpi Pradhan, MD

Editor of *How Healers Heal* Book

1

Heal a Doctor Mom to Heal a Nation: How One Physician's Lifestyle Journey Forever Changed Her Life, Her Parenting and Her Doctoring

Qadira Malika Ali, MD, MPH, FAAP, DipABLM

"My mission in life is not merely to survive, but to thrive; and to do so with some passion, some compassion, some humor, and some style."

— Maya Angelou

The slump in my back, as I walked out of my primary care physician's office, mirrored the almost perpetual defeated gait with which I found myself frequently ambulating around my own clinic these days. I had just left my annual physical exam with yet another refill of labetalol, a common medication used to treat high blood pressure. Despite half-hearted efforts to make lifestyle changes in my own life, I'd not yet been successful enough to wean off the medication. I felt a similar sense of impotence in my clinical practice as a primary care pediatrician—where I found myself increasingly frustrated with the lack of impact my brief visits had on patients and their parents.

In both my clinical practice and personal life, I was showing classic signs of burnout. I was increasingly emotionally exhausted, feeling the slip of disengagement, and wholly lacking in a sense of autonomy. How did I get to this place? And, more importantly, how did I get out of this place? The answers to these questions began with learning new paradigms for living. I learned what **not** to do as it related to my own health and well-being during residency, and I relearned exactly what **to** do to safeguard my health and that of my patients during my Lifestyle Medicine (LM) training.

During the most intense years of my clinical training during my pediatrics residency, I lived what I now call "the anti-lifestyle." Residency years are known to be the most grueling time of a young physician's training. On every level of being, one's mettle is tested—often in settings where support is limited.

From a physical standpoint, I was chronically sleep-deprived. While 80-hour workweek restrictions had been implemented prior to my residency, shifts could still be as long as 30 hours of expected wakefulness. Thirty hours of pagers alarming, nursing calls, patient emergencies, routine admissions and discharges, team rounding, and conference room didactics. Brief naps happened if I experienced "good luck" during such a long shift, but definitely could not be expected. Surviving these lengthier shifts meant relying on the ultra-processed foods that were stocked with titillating variety in the 24-hour hospital canteen. I often "treated" myself to a midnight ice cream sandwich or gummy bears. The sugar rush pacified me and became a crutch to get through long, challenging days and nights—of which there were many during my three years of residency.

From an emotional standpoint, I felt chronically stressed and over-whelmed by the pace of clinical activity, patient volume, the many life sacrifices expected to be made without complaint, and the lack of auton-omy and rigidity of my schedule. These stressors were compounded by the emotional weight of providing care for sometimes very sick children and working with their understandably stressed parents. As a newly married resident physician—just six weeks before starting residency—I had the additional stress of trying to establish a new family routine at home as I grappled with limited emotional bandwidth after exhausting days at work.

What happens to a person when the stressors are many, and the healthy coping skills are few? Health takes a major hit. By the time I graduated residency, I had gained 75 pounds, and I was grappling with a sense of malaise. As my occupational health physical would soon reveal, I also now had a new diagnosis of hypertension with a prescription to go along with it. I felt like I had aged much more than the mere three years that had passed.

It was in this state of flagging mental and physical health that I embarked upon my journey as a new attending pediatrician. I had dreamed of this milestone for many years, and to say that reality did not come close to delivering the dream would be an understatement. I soon found myself trapped reliving Groundhog Day as I sought to repeatedly im-part lifestyle advice to patients and parents who were on the verge of lifestyle-related chronic diseases, or worse, who already had them. I ques-tioned my impact. I questioned my approach. I questioned my own habits. The only thing I became certain of was that I was growing in-creasingly discontent with this type of clinical practice.

In a parallel experience of discontent, I was growing tired of feeling worn out in my personal life. Less than two years into being a full-time pediatrician, I birthed my first child—a beautiful baby girl. While some of my fatigue was expected as the parent of a young child, a significant portion of my exhaustion stemmed from my waning health. As the demands of my professional and personal responsibilities grew, I had not compensated by consistently filling my own metaphorical cup. And thus, the stress continued to pile on without a functional release valve. The feeling of burnout that had first taken hold during residency became even more entrenched, leaving me to daydream about what an escape from medicine could look like.

Before allowing myself to take action toward leaving clinical medicine, I knew that I had to do what I could to begin feeling better **now**. I had an initial goal of discontinuing my blood pressure medication under the care of my physician. In order to achieve this goal, I knew I had to get serious about weight loss. This goal led me to shift back to the largely unprocessed vegetarian diet of my childhood, re-engaging with more consistent physical activity, and finding stress-relief tools that I could utilize when short on time. Working intently on my physical health outside of work created more benefits both at home and in the clinic than there is space here to describe. One of the most significant revelations during this time of intense personal lifestyle revitalization was the symbiotic relationship between my own health practices and my approach to both doctoring and motherhood. Walking the healthy walk in my personal life strengthened my resolve to help facilitate healthy changes among those within my sphere of influence.

I felt a major shift in how I showed up for work after my health began to improve. I had slimmed down, weaned completely off of blood pressure medication, and found ways to make physical activity a routine part of my life. All of these positive changes influenced how I counseled patients and how motivated I was to help them establish healthier habits too. While pediatrics, as a field, is built upon preventive medicine and dosing out anticipatory guidance on varied topics related to holistic child health, it often felt like we were only skimming the surface of imparting just how essential healthy lifestyle habits were to maximizing whole family health. I yearned for support, for resources, and for a framework through which I could enhance my practice goal of helping kids and families truly thrive.

After one particularly unfulfilling day in the clinic, I decided to turn to Google for answers—despite my frequent exhortations to patients and parents not to do the same. While I was not looking for typical medical advice, I was looking for advice on how to practice medicine in a more holistic manner. I Googled "physician wellness" and "healthy lifestyle." After skimming the first few hits, I read a line that caught my eye: American College of Lifestyle Medicine (ACLM). After tumbling headfirst into the world of ACLM, I attended my first conference and got certified in 2019. I became forever changed as a physician, mother, and woman. I had finally found the language and framework to discuss and practice lifestyle-focused medicine. I had finally found a community of "like-minded" physicians.

While I had already created momentum in my life around establishing a healthy lifestyle, delving into the science of LM provided a roadmap to help me more holistically transform my everyday habits. Within a year and a half of beginning my lifestyle journey, I'd lost more than 50 pounds, was off blood pressure medication, ran 8Ks, and felt more empowered about my life and future in a way that I had not felt in any previous chapter. From my diet to stress management, each area of my lifestyle received a makeover for the better as I applied the science of LM to my own life.

From a dietary perspective, I shifted from a vegetarian diet that included high amounts of dairy and eggs to an exclusively plant-based diet built primarily on unprocessed food. This shift has helped me to maintain a significant weight loss and remain normotensive for the past four years and counting.

From a movement perspective, I found myself prioritizing my physical activity and intentionally looking for ways to add more natural movement to each day. For most of my adulthood, I'd struggled to find a consistent form of physical activity that I enjoyed. The emphasis on physical activity prompted me to rediscover my childhood love of cycling. I have relearned the importance of finding an activity that feels less like a chore and more like fun.

From a sleep perspective, I developed a deeper respect for the importance of daily restoration. While I still have imperfect sleep habits, understanding the science behind recommendations to prioritize high-quality sleep motivates me to be more mindful. I am now much more likely to "close up shop for the night" rather than push my limits of wakefulness in pursuit of higher "productivity." LM has given me science-backed permission to prioritize nightly rest.

From a stress management perspective, I began to actively experiment with healthy modes of coping with the ups and downs of life. Having a propensity toward feeling stressed has been part of my makeup for as long as I can remember. While some positive experiences of stress have been associated with goal achievement, I came to appreciate that chronically feeling "stressed out" presents significant mental and physical harm over the long term. LM motivated me to become much more intentional about integrating stress-relieving practices into my daily life. Whether I'm journaling or practicing meditation, or simply enjoying nature, I now diligently try to do at least one activity daily that grounds me. This single lifestyle pillar has been the glue that binds all the other six pillars together for me. If I am feeling a sense of balance, then that centeredness spills into all areas of my life.

From a healthy relationship perspective, I began to create more space for people in my life. As a recently divorced individual, understanding the science of loneliness in the context of this new chapter of singlehood has motivated me to nourish the many rich non-romantic relationships in my life. From childhood friends to siblings to coworkers, people do indeed "make the world go round." As a LM physician, I have been much more thoughtful about nurturing my relationships than I otherwise would have been.

One relationship, in particular, has both fueled and benefited from my lifestyle journey: the mother-daughter relationship. Once I became a mother, I felt that I had higher stakes to transform my health and lifestyle to set an example for my daughter. I took my responsibility as her first teacher seriously. As such, I wanted to ensure that among the many things I passed on to her were the tools for creating a healthy lifestyle. The critical importance of childhood as a time to establish norms motivated me to seek out every possible chance to teach her the "language of lifestyle." I have sought to make the various healthy habits we aspire to as commonplace as possible. LM has influenced my parenting style and decisions in a number of positive ways. From utilizing a mindful parenting approach to intertwining physical activity into our family culture, a healthy lifestyle lays at the foundation of our home. My daughter, at five years old, has basic cooking skills and a wonderful understanding of balanced healthy eating. She has a healthy foundation to build upon as she grows, and very few other things could make me more pleased as a mother.

My patients have also been beneficiaries of my LM journey. Before making LM changes in my personal life, I often felt like a fraud in clinic. I was not living the advice I was giving to my patients and their parents. Also, I did not have the lived experience to counsel on a healthy lifestyle in a practical way that integrates the complexity of a real, messy, busy life. How can parents actually prepare healthy quick meals? How can families squeeze in physical activity during a busy week? What does balance look like? Once I began making the effort to put these aspirations of a healthy lifestyle into practice, I could show up in a more authentic and useful way for my patients. I consolidated much of this learned and lived knowledge of practical Lifestyle Medicine into an entrepreneurial venture called *Sprouting Wellness*, which remains a virtual source of LM education for parents today.

After I completed my certification in Lifestyle Medicine, my approach to lifestyle counseling shifted dramatically to a more holistic, long-term view of healthy living. I shifted toward an approach that was less outcomes-focused and more processes-focused with the goal of laying the groundwork for sustainable and engrained healthy habits within families. I shifted my language in clinic regarding follow-up visit types from "weight checks" to "nutrition" or "lifestyle checks" as a way to emphasize the behaviors we were focused on versus a number on the scale. The science of plant-based nutrition also directs my dietary counseling for a number of common pediatric conditions—including eczema, constipation, obesity/overweight, and prediabetes.

Additionally, I noticed more subtle effects of my personal lifestyle change on my clinical practice. There was an uptick in implicit motivation I delivered to patients and families as they saw my changed physique—often sparking organic conversation about what I'd done and how I'd sustained it. I also noticed the connection between how I felt—both physically and emotionally—with my experience of practicing medicine. My sense of resilience at work was boosted as I carved out time to take good care of myself.

To summarize all of what I've shared thus far: Lifestyle Medicine has been transformative to every domain of my personal and professional life. Given the current health landscape and bleak projections for ever-worsening lifestyle-related chronic diseases among children and adults, I wholeheartedly believe that Lifestyle Medicine represents the future of medicine. The research is clear that doctors are not unidimensional and that our personal lifestyle habits impact our doctoring. Therefore, doctors *and* patients need Lifestyle Medicine. The movement of Lifestyle Medicine is growing and expanding its reach into how doctors are trained. Beyond integrating LM into medical training at all levels, the field of Lifestyle Medicine must doggedly pursue how this life-saving approach may be a source of healing for all communities—especially medically underserved and racially minoritized groups experiencing deep health inequities. Lifestyle Medicine may help to achieve health equity as its principles can be adapted to be culturally relevant across diverse communities. Through LM advocacy, my clinical practice, and *Sprouting Wellness*, I strive to build healthier future generations—one child, family, and community at a time.

This chapter is dedicated to my sparkling daughter, Zora, who reminds me daily to breathe, have fun, and never stop growing.

About Dr. Qadira Malika Ali, MD, MPH, FAAP, DiplABLM

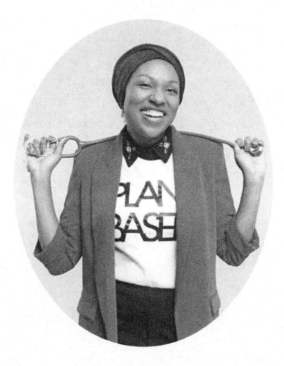

Dr. Qadira M. Ali is a board-certified pediatrician, certified lifestyle medicine physician and clinical assistant professor of pediatrics. Dr. Ali practices as a primary care pediatrician at Children's National Hospital. She is also the founder/CEO of Sprouting Wellness, a lifestyle medicine platform for families that focuses on healthful lifestyle habits, including plant-based nutrition, movement, and mindfulness. Dr. Ali graduated from the University of Maryland School of Medicine (M.D.) and Johns Hopkins Bloomberg School of Public Health (M.P.H.) with a focus on food systems, equity, and health disparities. Dr. Ali completed a pediatrics residency at Children's National Hospital with a training focus on historically underserved populations. She is certified in plant-based nutrition from eCornell and the T. Colin Campbell Center for Nutrition Studies.

Dr. Ali serves as a public health and lifestyle medicine expert advisor to communities, organizations, and industry. Dr. Ali is an active member of the American College of Lifestyle Medicine (ACLM) and co-chair of ACLM's Health Equity Achieved through Lifestyle Medicine Initiative. She also serves on the Board of Directors for the Plant-Based Prevention of Disease nonprofit. Dr. Ali was selected as the inaugural Physician Wellness Lead for the division of primary care pediatrics at Children's National Hospital. In 2019, she founded the Hyattsville, MD chapter of Walk With A Doc. Dr. Ali lives in Maryland with her family. In her free time, she enjoys writing, cycling, hiking, traveling, and reading.

Sprouting Wellness: https://www.sproutingwellness.com/about

Instagram: https://www.instagram.com/sproutingwellnessmd/

Watch an interview with the co-author:

Co-Author spotlight
DR. QADIRA MALIKA ALI

Scan Me

2

Breaking Generational Medical History

Shruthi Chandrashekhar, MD, DipABOM, DipABLM

"Believe in yourself and all that you are. Know that there is something inside of you that is greater than any obstacle."
— Christian D. Larson

I'm reflecting on my story sitting in my lifestyle and obesity medicine clinic . . . feels surreal. How did I get here, and why did I get here?

It wasn't an aha moment. Although I have had my fair share of struggles in life from childhood to medical school, my most concerning childhood memory involves struggling with my dad's poor health due to coronary heart disease. He was only 32 years old when he had his first heart attack! Yup, younger than my age now. What did they do back then for him? . . . No lifestyle changes . . . just saying to be careful. It was such a reset in our lives. My brother had just been born, and we all were scared of losing my dad any day. Fortunately, he is now 66 years old and, touch wood, after cardiac bypass surgery at the mere age of 44 and again stents at age 64, he is ok for now. With his multiple issues on and off, the journey has been nothing less than scary. Regarding our prior generations, all my grandfathers died by the age of 38–44 years old. I have never met my grandfathers.

With my family history, I was naturally interested in cardiology. But while I was exploring other fields during my residency, I just wasn't convinced that my life's calling was in formal cardiology training. I was always interested in the preventive side of medicine, so I continued to explore all areas of medicine, and I chose to begin working as a hospitalist, where I saw the most complex of patients. At this phase of my life, this was where my calling was, as I saw hundreds of patients with chronic diseases who were treated for their condition, but no one was addressing their lifestyle or looking into the possibility of reversal of their condition.

Ironically, I also have PCOS, which runs in my family and is a significant disease burden. When I was younger, I was told that oral contraceptive pills were the only effective treatment for this condition, but lifestyle was not addressed, which I now know to be an effective treatment.

While I practiced hospital medicine, I completely changed my lifestyle from healthy to one of convenience. I was eating a lot of takeout food as I had no time or energy to cook for myself. My PCOS got worse, which affected my energy and my sleep. I can say I was hardly thriving but continued with my lifestyle. After a few years of this lifestyle, we decided to have a baby. With PCOS, conceiving was a challenge. Pregnancy came with its challenges, as I had to be on insulin shots and keep a close check on my sugars for the rest of my pregnancy. Pregnancy made me think about if there was something else I could have done differently in my journey toward my first baby boy.

The following two years held more challenges with a growing child, and I was fortunate to have another child. I was still trying to balance it all but hardly succeeding. I couldn't lose the weight I gained this time around. I needed to be on insulin shots like my prior pregnancy. I managed somehow, but afterward, I was left with extra weight, extra responsibilities, and struggling to balance my life as a doctor and wife, and now I was a full-blown diabetic. I felt ashamed that, being a physician, I couldn't take care of myself, and I couldn't take care of my eating or medicines like I was able to when I was pregnant. This time wasn't like a 9-month drill, but an uncertain timeline and unknown endpoint. I started to try the "diabetic diet," . . . and things got worse. To sum up my situation, I was a 38-year-old with uncontrolled diabetes, my HbA1c numbers in the 8s, and an overweight physician on four different meds for diabetes. I felt defeated!

As my PCOS flared over the next few months, I had become severely anemic. I had to call EMS when I developed chest pain resulting from severe anemia. I had my babies with me, one four-year-old and another hardly six months old, both looking at the EMS crew coming into our home as I was about to be taken to the ER. I remember looking from the stretcher at my son's face . . . it scared me. At the hospital, I was diagnosed with severe anemia and coronary spasms. I needed a blood transfusion, and I was started on medications for my heart. I spent a night in the same hospital room where I had treated so many patients, feeling crushed to be in this situation. I didn't want to accept the course of my condition and feel powerless. I knew I needed to change. The scare of almost having a heart attack and being diagnosed with a heart condition at such a young age caused me to panic, especially with two small children who depended on me.

I continued to focus on eating a keto diet or whatever low-carb food I could and squeezed in some exercise. I didn't see any changes. Serendipitously, this is when one of my colleagues, Dr. Shilpi Pradhan, mentioned that she is certified in Lifestyle Medicine (LM). The new field piqued my interest. I checked it out, and I was curious and joined the special interest group of physicians in the field of LM.

"Synergy and serendipity often play a big part in medical and scientific advances."

— Julie Bishop

I was looking to learn for myself. I was looking to heal from within, something for me, more than for patient care. However, when I joined their group and started to be a part of the conversation, I remember following one of the LM physician's personal blogs, and I started making changes to my diet and lifestyle. As I began to learn more, over the next 10 months, I changed my cooking technique. Following the other pillars of health, I started to notice my energy getting better, my blood sugars, though not perfect, were improving, and my sleep was improving. That is when I decided to become certified and signed up for LM board certification. I met some incredible fellow colleagues who made such an impact on their patients and communities. They became my inspiration, and my patients and my family were my motivation. Our entire family life improved, including our nutrition and relationships within our family.

After seeing how much LM has impacted my life, I want to empower my patients to take control, utilize the knowledge of the six pillars of health, especially those which matter to them the most, and change. I want them not to feel defeated and accept fate as my father was guided to do decades ago. I want them to know their health is in their control. I believe LM is the way future medical practice is headed for preventing and treating patients in all aspects of their lives.

While continuing to practice hospital medicine, I've been fortunate to join my dream Obesity and Lifestyle Medicine clinic, called ZoeStyle Medicine, to help patients achieve their goals. Several patients have given me back my purpose and passion for medicine through practicing lifestyle medicine. Their efforts in applying and practicing lifestyle changes have inspired and renewed my passion for the field. One patient, who was socio-economically disadvantaged and had depression due to her physical health and weight, started attending our weekly group coaching and eventually saw me for a consultation. Although she had limited resources, she was motivated and made considerable strides in improving her health within two months, including losing 15 lbs, normalizing her BP, improving her baseline energy, and eliminating her shortness of breath. She is one of many patients who inspire me and who

I admire for their strength and dedication. My team and I are committed to helping patients discover lifestyle changes, and they are committed to making them. We are a team in improving their health, and it is simply transformative and magical.

———◆◇◆———

I dedicate this chapter to my husband (Dr. Santhosh Kumar), who has been immensely supportive on this journey of health in every crazy possible way I could ask for. Also, to my mom and dad and my two boys, who I need to live well for.

———◆◇◆———

About Dr. Shruthi Chandrashekhar, MD, DipABOM, DipABLM

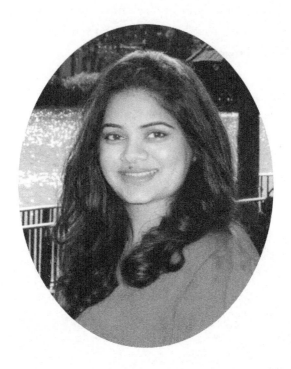

Dr. Shruthi Chandrashekhar is a triple board-certified physician with expertise in Internal Medicine, Obesity Medicine, and Lifestyle Medicine. Understanding lifestyle factors in health and disease has long been an interest. After completing medical school in India, she graduated from Columbia University's St. Luke's-Roosevelt residency program in NYC, where she was involved in a special project on nutrition and obesity. Upon completing her residency, she came to Virginia, where she has been a hospital medicine physician for the last several years while concurrently pursuing her certifications in Obesity and Lifestyle Medicine. Dr. Chandrashekhar understands the challenges that one faces as a patient with chronic conditions. She comes to ZoeStyle Medicine with the right knowledge and understanding of the pathways to healing and is here to support and recommend the best treatment to achieve one's goals. She joins a select few physicians across the country with such expertise and would like to make a significant impact on her patients and community.

Website: https://zoerva.com/zoestyle-medicine/

<u>Watch an interview with the co-author:</u>

Co-Author spotlight
DR. SHRUTHI
CHANDRASHEKHAR

Scan Me

3

A Timely Gift Turns into a Gift of Time

Cherie Chu, MD, FAAP, DipABLM

"We have a hard time putting ourselves on our own priority list, let alone at the top of it. And that's what happens when it comes to our health as women. We are so busy giving and doing for others that we almost feel guilty to take that time out for ourselves."

— Michelle Obama

Lifestyle Medicine found me long before I found it. Years ago, a colleague told me about a conference at the Culinary Institute of America called *Healthy Kitchens Healthy Lives,* and I thought, "Good food and CME? I'm in." Far from my days of scrounging for food in the resident's lounge, I looked forward to a conference where I got to eat delicious food to my heart's content. Little did I know this would be the inflection point where my life would change forever.

Before this, I was a bad cook (or at least I believed I was). Meals put together with pre-made or frozen food were a staple in my home. When I learned about the tremendous impact of food on our health at the conference, I decided I needed to learn to cook. I wanted something better for my kids, my husband, and for myself.

I started cooking more often using the skills I learned at the conference. Blanch vegetables? Check. Chop onions? Check. With practice, I developed the confidence to cook more meals from scratch. My kids liked to help and would often chomp on the chopped vegetables while we cooked together. Their culinary curiosity normalized eating vegetables for them, which made my job of feeding them easier. I noticed I felt better when I ate better, but it wasn't until I discovered Lifestyle Medicine (LM) a few years later that everything seemed to click.

Lifestyle Medicine fell in my lap at exactly the time I needed it most. It all started when I lost my mom to cancer and gave birth to twins in the span of less than a year. Navigating motherhood while simultaneously grieving the loss of my mother was challenging both physically and emotionally. My husband supported me in so many ways, yet I often found myself drowning in a sea of diapers and burp cloths, wishing I could pick up the phone to hear her voice at the other end.

To say I was overwhelmed and exhausted is an understatement. Despite my husband's best efforts to give me the space he knew I needed to take care of me, I put myself on the back burner as I busied myself with my roles as a pediatrician and a mom. I loved my job, but trying to work as if I didn't have children and be a mom as if I didn't have a job quickly led to burnout. I knew I couldn't continue feeling the way I was feeling, and this is what triggered me to go searching for a different path. It was on this path where I found Lifestyle Medicine.

The moment I learned about Lifestyle Medicine, I was so sure it was the perfect fit that I immediately pursued board certification. LM encourages healthcare practitioners to "walk the walk" in their own lives to effectively teach our patients. So that is what I did. I made sleep, exercise, and mindfulness a priority in addition to the changes I had already made to my eating habits, and I began to feel more balanced. I was able to concentrate better, improving my efficiency at work and giving me more time at the end of each day. I felt like I was getting my life back.

Lifestyle Medicine gave me a new fulfilling way of practicing medicine.

I had always given my patients the standard "Eat your vegetables and exercise" talk with little to no uptake prior to becoming a LM doctor. It was the coaching education from the LM coursework that taught me how to help patients to effect change for themselves. When I utilized this approach, I started seeing a real impact on my patients' lives. There's nothing like a parent telling you their child is "a different person" because of something you taught them. As I began seeing similar results over and over again, I felt a new sense of purpose and enjoyment in my medical practice.

I was so inspired by the changes I saw in myself and my patients that I joined a team of like-minded physicians in my medical group to develop a LM curriculum to teach our colleagues about the six pillars of LM. We cooked together virtually and taught a LM implementation series. We were delighted to see our physician colleagues change their own lives and, in some cases, the lives of their family members too. It was exciting to imagine the potentially exponential level of impact they would bring to their patients.

It became my mission to share LM beyond the exam room. I started an educational pediatric lifestyle medicine website called Wellness Pediatrician because I wanted to empower both parents and healthcare practitioners to teach children healthy habits beginning in early childhood. I provide teaching tools and strategies to give them the support they need. Can you imagine if we could teach a whole generation of children that eating the colors of the rainbow every day is normal? I want to empower the next generation to grow up well and stay well.

In many ways, I feel my journey into Lifestyle Medicine and the outcome of its implementation is the legacy my mom gave to me. Arising from the emptiness of my own early motherhood, I landed on a path leading me to flourish personally and professionally. LM gave me a renewed sense of enjoyment in medicine, improved health for my family and myself, and empowered me to teach children to live a healthy lifestyle right from the start. I will be forever grateful to my mom, not just for the life that she gave me but for the life she continues to give me every day.

———◄○►———

Dedicated to my loving husband, who builds the foundation on which our wins are possible, and to my kids, whose creativity and curiosity inspire me every day. You are my why for everything I do, and I am so grateful for your selfless love and support.

To my mom - Our time together was too short and I miss you deeply. Thank you for everything you and Dad sacrificed to give me and my family this life.

———◄○►———

About Dr. Cherie Chu, MD, FAAP, DipABLM

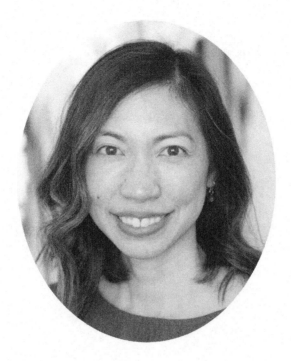

Dr. Cherie Chu is board certified in Pediatrics and Lifestyle Medicine and practices outpatient pediatrics at Sharp Rees-Stealy Medical Group in San Diego, CA. She is the founder of Wellness Pediatrician, a Pediatric Lifestyle Medicine educational website dedicated to helping children grow up with healthy lifestyle habits. She is also the founder of Doctor Moms Lounge, a membership designed to help women physicians take the busywork out of "momming," so they have time for what matters to them most.

WELLNESS PEDIATRICIAN

Website: https://www.wellnesspediatrician.com/

Instagram: https://www.instagram.com/wellnesspediatrician/

DOCTOR MOMS LOUNGE

Website: https://doctormomslounge.com/

Instagram: https://www.instagram.com/doctormomslounge/

<u>Watch an interview with the co-author:</u>

Co-Author spotlight
DR. CHERIE CHU

4

Tying It All Together: LM Fulfills All of This Physician's Career Aspirations

Nupur Garg, MD, DipABLM

"The journey of a thousand miles begins with one step."
— Lao Tzu, circa 400 BCE

My story begins in ancient India, long before I was born. South Asian cultures tend to have an aspirational relationship with the past, which has always intrigued me. Though I self-identify as an early adopter when it comes to new technology, ancient ideas for health and wellness have enough value to modern societies that they continue to be widely practiced. Our parents and family members would teach us yoga and meditation here and there throughout our childhood as they practiced. This practical knowledge was passed down through generational wisdom long before Western medicine studied these practices and found they were objectively beneficial.

Another age-old cultural tradition that piqued my intrigue is the consumption and benefits of bitter vegetables and certain spices known to treat diseases now but used preventively by our ancestors. Massage therapy, breathing exercises, the importance of community, maintaining purpose, sleeping practices, commitment to a life partner . . . it was all so prescribed in ancient South Asian culture in a way that almost negates free will. Therefore, human nature should have rejected it, especially after so long. Yet, what was almost equally perplexing was that almost all of Indian society still maintained at least an aspirational notion toward this culture. How has it been handed down from generation to generation over millennia in such a neatly packaged manner, covering almost all aspects of health and wellness?

Excitingly, South Asian culture is not unique. Growing up in the USA, I loved learning about other cultures, not just from literature where I could better understand the historical influences of the various cultural norms over the years. I also felt privileged to experience diverse cultures through the people I met. Millennial-old knowledge passed down in the form of cultural norms about healthy lifestyles exists in almost all corners of the world. It's also not all the same, which makes sense because of environmental influences on our lifestyles, but it has always fascinated me that there is considerable overlap.

In the absence of high-power microscopy, I suppose that the predominant manner in which these practices are maintained is through faith. One thing I've learned about faith is that it does not exist without stories. Stories are engaging, memorable, fun, and full of lessons. In South Asian culture, countless stories helped to deliver ancient messages through the generations.

Importantly, society has evolved to need more than just faith when it comes to choices about lifestyles. To forego indulgences, we need proof that our choice will result in a happier future self. We *need* proof now because we can *have* proof now. Long gone are the days of leeches and home-based apothecaries. Evidence-based medicine is the standard of care. As a physician, in some ways, it is both our weapon and our shield. We will never be faulted for following the guidelines if, at the time which we followed them, that was the scientific 'truth' with the information we had. But for anyone following closely, these guidelines are constantly changing. Sometimes, we change practices in a matter of months. This raises the natural question: If something was proven in science, why would it ever change? Also, if something was never proven, does that mean it is not valid?

The science of medicine is, in fact, not a perfect science. It is not like the science of physics, math, chemistry, or biology, especially if our measurements are subjective (how someone feels, how much pain someone is in, how much energy someone has) rather than objective. Most physicians agree that the best type of evidence that can exist in medicine is called a double-blind, randomized, controlled trial. That means that neither the research participants nor the researchers know who is getting the intervention; the intervention is given to the participants at random, and there is a group of people who did not receive the intervention (aka control group). Often, the studies are done by averaging across ages from 18–65+ and across genders, ethnicities, and comorbidities. This study design is meant to find treatments for diseases like infections, organ dysfunction, or cancer. But the problem is that specific responses to interventions can be very individual. For example, cancer trials may have shown that a potential treatment cured cancer in one person but failed in the other ten people in the trial, and, therefore, it was considered a failure using the gold standard methodology of science. A more important inquiry might be, can we determine which specific type of people this therapy might work for? This is the basis for personalized medicine, which is more in line with how I view the scientific field of medicine.

Furthermore, the studies that do show evidence under the gold standard methodology of randomized, double-blinded, controlled trials are not fool-proof. At MIT, I took a class taught by two Nobel laureates. It was a seminar class, and each week, each student would get assigned one of the foundational papers in developmental biology, and their task would be to tear it apart. These were papers upon which theories upon theories have been tested and proven, and yet each week, we would rip it to shreds—and it was completely exhilarating. By the end of every class, I'd always be humbled at all the critiques I hadn't thought of. Over time, I became skilled at reading research papers from such a critical lens. Even after studies pass through all of our critiques and get accepted for publication, they still have biases and limitations. Almost nothing in medical science is ever set in stone.

In medicine, our foundational knowledge is based on biology in theory but has proven to be evidence-based using statistics. This is because, whereas biology research happens in a lab, where everything from the temperature and humidity of the room to the exact timing and quantity of compounds can be controlled, clinical medicine happens in the real world, which is far from the controlled environment of a lab. Even things we can theoretically control, like medication dosages, are not precise. Pharmaceutical factories are allowed to have a certain margin of error in manufacturing medications that might lead to significant variability if the medication dosages are in micrograms, like certain thyroid medications. All that said, I think some amount of information is obtained through each study that is done, even studies that are not "successful."

Even if research studies indicate a particular intervention to be successful, the healthcare system is not always set up to incentivize that practice. Many people working in healthcare are disillusioned by the perverse incentives of the system. In fact, some "rules" that the system dictates we follow are contrary to what might be best for patient care. Instead, the healthcare system is designed to keep maximized profits at the forefront of priorities. Some companies with the highest profits in the country are pharmaceutical companies, retail pharmacies, insurance companies, and large hospital systems. What often means better patient care means fewer profits for these industries. There are new programs just starting called value-based care models, which are helping to align some of the incentives toward optimal patient health outcomes.

Armed with my intrigue of generational, multicultural health and wellness advice, a healthy dose of wariness of the claims of medical "research" and "best practices," and an attitude of being a lifelong learner, I was ready to hear about a new field in medicine that was focused on evidence-based healthy lifestyle recommendations for the prevention and treatment of chronic diseases. My introduction to Lifestyle Medicine (LM) began while researching healthy ways to raise my young family. My children are vegan, and I, myself not having been raised on a vegan diet, wanted to learn all the evidence that existed on plant-based, healthy diets for kids. To be honest, I really did not expect to find that much. Little did I realize that the foundational research in LM is several decades old, and so much has been studied in so many realms. Though I, too, absolutely loved learning through informal mechanisms, just as a non-medical consumer of podcasts and articles, once I learned that there was a LM curriculum with a textbook and certification process, I signed up immediately.

Initially, I pursued LM certification with no idea I would eventually transition into practicing the field as my primary specialty. I simply thought that the structure of the certification program would be best in terms of consuming all the existing evidence for healthy lifestyle choices. I was pregnant with my second child when I started, and she was a toddler when I finished. Life was busy! I loved every minute. I wanted to learn everything I could. I wanted to know the quality of evidence for the recommendations and what was yet to be determined. I reproduced the material in many different formats, including flashcards that I'd take with me on walks with my kids and tables and diagrams that I used to review material with colleagues in a study group we had formed. Eventually, these study buddies and I published our tables in a book called: _Guidebook to Ace the Lifestyle Medicine Boards_, which I continually reference in my LM practice.

During this time, a documentary promoting plant-based nutrition came out on Netflix and was very popular among my friends. I became a sort-of fact checker for them, and through this experience, I also learned what sort of questions mattered most to people when considering a major lifestyle change. Also, now becoming plant-based or plant-forward was no longer such a completely wild idea. I started using my knowledge and experience in coaching my friends in my practice in the Emergency Department (ED). I realized that I was good at explaining LM to people and patients, and they were listening to me.

At a LM conference, one physician talked about how he learned so much from the sales and marketing industry that has helped him support his patients and reach their outcome goals. He said the two most important messages were: 1. Manage your own emotions, and 2. Manage your patients' emotions. We, as humans, are very good at knowing when we are being sold something and we don't like it. We have a natural distrust for something too salesy. I loved this message because I believe that the culture of medicine in the US has, at times, been too paternalistic. It often doesn't respect one's agency enough or consider their individuality enough.

Having this perspective already made it easy for me to let go of my personal ego or ownership over patients' choices and instead empathize with each patient and their personal situation. The fact that we are all born into a certain way of life that ultimately influences how we think and behave is one way in which we are all connected. Understanding people through their own lens of themselves is so essential for my work as a LM physician.

Even so, it was nerve-wracking the first few times I stood in front of a patient in the ED and told them to eat more vegetables. I remember one of the first patients I introduced LM to was a patient who felt like every time he ate take-out Chinese food, he'd have his stroke symptoms again and end up in the ED again. Another one of my patients felt he should be able to take a sufficient amount of insulin and eat whatever he wanted. A third patient was found to have kidney failure, and I wanted to admit him, but he refused. Finally, he said, "I know I've been unhealthy recently, but I can fix it. I will start exercising, and just tell me exactly what to eat, and I'll eat it." These were just a few patients that I remember, but there were more. I realized these patients probably have been here all along asking me for input on their lifestyle, and I just never registered it. The more I knew about LM, the more patients I'd find that were receptive to hearing about it. I realized patients wanted this—they *have been* wanting it. It was me who didn't know enough before. Furthermore, physicians want to know this.

After my shift was over, I spent 30 minutes at a time counseling patients about healthy lifestyle choices. They were always so appreciative, and I also loved doing it. Ultimately, I realized I wanted to have some semblance of a practice in LM. So, I contacted my employer and asked to start a clinic in LM. They put me in charge of a LM working group, and I gave a few talks about LM to physicians. After six months, I realized it would be years before I could practice LM through the hospital system, so I opened up my own clinic. A few months later, I left my employed position in the ED to work in my LM clinic full-time.

One thing I love about LM is that it requires each practicing LM physician to be on their own action plan toward adopting LM practices. At first, it seemed a little overbearing, but there is 'evidence' for it! Physicians who have unhealthy lifestyles are less likely to discuss healthy lifestyle choices with their patients. Also, we are encouraged to pull from our personal journeys to help patients make the prescribed changes. Having a personal action plan fits my personality as a life-long learner and as someone who is always trying to improve. As I like to tell my patients: *Every step in the right direction is a step away from the wrong one.*

One concept I always try to remember is that not every person's goal is the same. LM strives to help each person sustain a disease-free and lengthy life, but each of us has other additional aspects we want to enjoy in our lives, including perhaps a certain kind of food, custom, comfort, or other indulgences. With LM, we are now able to make our choices with full knowledge of the effects on our health, which can be liberating in a way and allow us to enjoy our choices even more.

One of my most challenging changes was giving up sugar. It took me several attempts, and each relapse came with a binge period. That said, each attempt mattered and got me closer to my goal. With my most recent and final attempt, I had been eating sugar approximately ten times per day. I quit cold turkey and had such terrible withdrawal symptoms that I couldn't sleep. My headache only lightened up after I ate half a banana. On this final quit attempt, my husband supported me immensely. He bought me sugar-free products to replace the trigger products I usually relapsed with (chocolate chips) and made all his recipes with sugar replacements. I eventually stopped needing the sugar replacements. I currently eat sugar five times per year—on each of my family member's birthdays and Thanksgiving. After giving up sugar, I felt almost immediately healthier. It was like night and day in terms of the frequency of illnesses, the severity of illnesses, and general energy. I also lost weight even though I felt I was eating an increased volume of food. I waited an entire year before trying to make another lifestyle change. Currently, I'm working on cutting out fried foods!

Compared to cutting out bad habits, adding in good habits presents less of a mental challenge and more of a logistic challenge. There never seem to be enough hours in a day. To assist with this problem, I turned to the idea of downshifting, another concept I learned about in LM. Downshifting involves choosing to simplify one's life, either through committing to less or working less, in order to achieve a better quality of life. Contrary to how I was raised, I chose to work less and lower my standard of living to have a better quality of life. It was a painful choice to make, and now my only regret is not doing it sooner.

One common theme I've seen brought up among many LM physicians is that it is much more complicated than we thought to change the mindset of our closest family members. For all the people I'd love to see change the most because of how much I care about them, it is almost a complete non-starter. After a particularly negative interaction where I made my father feel like a terrible husband for wanting to share a tasty, sweet dish with his wife (my mother) on a family vacation, I gave up on the unsolicited advice. Instead, I invited my family members to join a chat group in which I discuss one aspect of health and wellness per month.

LM is completely embedded into my being and soul. However, setting up my own clinic presented its own challenges. First, I had to develop a complementary business model, and I instinctively tried to choose something other than fee-for-service. I did not want to be incentivized to hope people would be sick. Instead, I learned about a model called Direct Primary Care (DPC), and I fell in love with it. DPC is a subscription-based primary care model that removes the middlemen from the relationship between the physician and the patient for all outpatient care needs. It replaces these with benefits which include wholesale pricing of meds, labs at <10% insurance rates, and imaging starting at $50 for X-rays, including the interpretation and facility fees. Patients may or may not have insurance. I personally do not have commercial health insurance. I have a health cost share plan instead, which covers potential hospital care. Either way, patients pay a monthly fee that gives them unlimited access to the DPC physician through any mode of communication they want. (Note: DPC clinics are all different.)

As an EM physician, one of my major "value-adds" to patients is keeping my patients out of the ED as much as possible. I have an ultrasound, IV hydration, UTI testing, strep throat testing, laceration repair, earwax removal, wound care, foreign body removal, and several other procedures accessible from my clinic, including after business hours, and there is no additional fee for anything. I also provide a free whole food plant-based cooking class in my teaching kitchen each month and an activity class at one of the nearby community locations each month (e.g., tai chi or chair yoga). I tell my patients, "I believe in skill power over willpower." Not everything should be hard, and if I can fill in knowledge gaps or skills to make change easier, then I will. I love being a one-stop shop for my patients. We have an "old-school" patient-doctor relationship but with modern medicine. I am expanding my teaching with social media and have high-yield educational videos on YouTube—my patients love it!

I always tell people that I set up my practice the way I imagine healthcare should be delivered. I believe the current healthcare system is lacking in many ways, and there are lots of opportunities to innovate. On the other hand, I also don't want to walk into a clinic and have a machine provide my primary care entirely and I never see a person. My ideal healthcare system maximizes the impact of the patient-doctor relationship, and I, as the doctor, stay the most up-to-date with my knowledge base and skills using as many tools as I can that can save my patients' money in addition to their health.

Even with my current DPC practice, I have a wish list of ideal tools that would help me take better care of my patients. One example is for administering asynchronous validated screening tools. The American College of Lifestyle Medicine employs dozens of helpful screening tools but using them all with the current healthcare system is a daunting task for a solo provider because they are typically administered in person and scored manually. They all help with early disease detection and prevention, though. It turns out I am actually well-positioned to provide a solution for this particular problem.

Before learning about LM, I already had an app called **Caspia** in the Apple iOS store that helps patients stay connected with their health data, including pulling in Apple Health and MyChart data. This app grew out of a need with my parents being unable to keep up with their health information despite being physicians themselves. Caspia allows users to take multimedia notes and track symptoms and medications. The stored data is searchable and more user-friendly than the MyChart or Apple Health platforms. With my new interest in LM and the need for the completion of screening tools, I thought, why not send my patients these screening tools through the app? They could answer on their own time, and the app would automatically score it and then send me the results. So, I formed a startup called Pro-Patient Tech (PPT) with this specific goal in mind. PPT's mission is to improve patients' health outcomes by using technology to assist physicians. So far, we have had amazing feedback from LM physicians. We have even been able to add more features, like trending vital signs and lab results and sending automatic reminders for screening tests (e.g., colonoscopy).

The culmination of my birth circumstances, passions, interests, intellect, life experiences, and current stage in life has made LM such a perfect fit for me. LM has changed my life in so many different ways, and I can't wait to see how it continues to evolve. In sharing my story, I hope some part of it resonates with others and helps them change their life with LM as much as it has changed mine.

This chapter is dedicated to the many people who have been my constant source of inspiration in my personal journey, including all of my loved ones and also my patients. Because of each of you, I'm able to do what I love and love what I do.

About Dr. Nupur Garg, MD, DipABLM

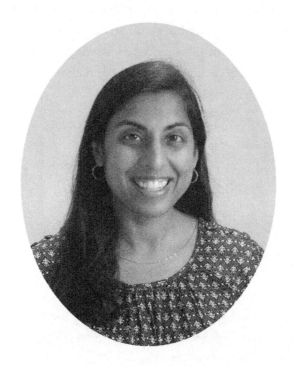

Dr. Nupur Garg is a dual board-certified practicing Lifestyle Medicine physician with a clinic called "Lifestyle and Family Medicine" near New Haven, CT. She completed her undergraduate education at MIT, went to Yale for Medical School, and did her residency at Mount Sinai in NYC. She has won numerous awards in research, entrepreneurship, and community building. She lives with her husband and two young children.

Dr. Garg's book on Lifestyle Medicine:

Garg, N., Kuhl, S., & Lee, J. (2022). *Guidebook to Ace the Lifestyle Medicine Boards.*

Website: https://www.lifestyleandfamilymedicine.com/

Instagram: https://www.instagram.com/ctlifestylemd/

YouTube: https://www.youtube.com/@nupurgargmd8757

Watch an interview with the co-author:

Co-Author spotlight

DR. NUPUR GARG

Scan Me

5

Finding Purpose: Making This Life a Journey of Service

Prachi Garodia, MD, ABIM, ABIHM, DipABLM, DipAyu, NBC-HWC

"Health is a dynamic state of balance of the physical, mental, emotional, and spiritual well-being; a state of harmony within yourself, your actions, the environment, nature, and the whole universe."

— Dr. Prachi Garodia

I clearly remember the shimmer of grateful tears in my paraplegic patient's eyes, who had managed to release around 30 lbs of weight over six months. She came in for an unexpected thank-you visit. I also recalled her desperation approximately seven months ago when I met her for the first time. Her life had taken a serious downward spiral a year before we met when she fractured several cervical vertebrae, severing her spinal cord during what had started as another adventure-filled day of her fun-filled life of kiteboarding on the weekends in Columbia Gorge in the beautiful Pacific Northwest.

During our second meeting, she tearfully shared her frustration about her inability to lose weight now that she was paralyzed and unable to move her limbs. She was living life lying in bed with her caregivers' periodic turning of her body. She also needed an attendant for all her activities of daily living, from turning in bed to taking a bath, dressing, eating, and sitting in a wheelchair. She went from being an extremely active and vibrant young woman to being completely bedridden. In addition, she was now suffering from obesity, not only due to immobility but more so due to highly processed, nutrient-deficient foods being provided to her by her long-term care residential facility.

Her blood pressure (BP) was going up, and her facility wanted to start her on BP medications. Her goal was to lose some of the extra weight which caused her high BP. She also wanted to feel lighter in her body to help her mobility despite being bed-bound. She shared her goals, and we formed a plan together with her aspirations for her health in mind using the SMART (Specific, Measurable, Action-Oriented/Achievable, Relevant, Time-Bound) goals strategy [1]. Next, I shared Lifestyle Medicine (LM) and Integrative Medicine (IM) tips for restoring her health and well-being, including stress management techniques, deep abdominal breathing, and sleep optimization. She eagerly took the after-visit summary with my detailed instructions on the six pillars of LM. She told me she would display it in several places in her room as a constant reminder to her and her caregivers.

We scheduled a telephone follow-up in two weeks to answer any questions and clarify her plan. I was amazed at her determination to follow the instructions to the hilt. At her three-month telephone visit, she reported she had been dutifully following most of the recommendations and had started seeing improvement in her health by the third week (which, of course, did not include any physical activity due to her paraplegia). She noticed her body releasing excess weight, her sleep getting better, and her moods being uplifted. She was much more cheerful. Her nurses reported her BP consistently within normal range by the second month after following the LM/IM recommendations. I welcomed her to contact me with any barriers, challenges, or questions that arose in the next few months, but I did not hear from her.

At her six-month surprise in-person visit, I was overjoyed to see a transformed, cheerful person smiling ear to ear in her wheeled bed. She had tears of gratitude flowing down her cheeks while we talked about her journey of health recovery. Hearing about her success brought me immense professional satisfaction and appreciation. The universe's goals for my professional duty and her determination to follow her dreams and goals for her health were in harmony.

We celebrated her big win in the clinic by sharing her story with the rest of her clinical team and front desk staff. She requested a photo with all of us which we happily obliged after she was transferred to the wheelchair from being bed-bound. She continued to lose weight gradually over the next several months. She was ecstatic to finally reach her pre-accident baseline weight, utilizing the simple but powerful lifestyle-based tips and techniques we continued to share.

This experience re-established my faith in the power of healing potential of the self and the power of the mind. Despite her significant limitation of mobility, she could accomplish what she wanted for herself with true grit and determination and staying true to her passion and goals.

> *"If you restore balance in your own self, you will be contributing immensely to the healing of the world."*
> — Deepak Chopra, MD

Now, a little bit about my own journey of healing . . .

Growing up, I was an intuitive and empathic child. I automatically drew toward myself anybody suffering, regardless of the species, whether it be a bird, a four-legged animal, or a fellow human being. From my earliest childhood memories, I remember nurturing the lost baby birds who had fallen from their nests while trying their maiden flight and sheltering and adopting the stray puppies who had somehow gotten separated from their moms and were whimpering soulfully on the streets.

I have always felt deeply connected to nature, which offers unlimited recharging energy to all beings. We grew up in an open, natural space, playing with bugs, squirrels, birds, and other animals around us and enjoying their company. We were also nourished with fresh home-cooked meals three times daily, prepared by our mother with endless love, with the use of seasonal herbs and spices aligned with the intelligence of nature passed down through generations. In addition, we utilized integrative modalities like homeopathy, Ayurveda, and yoga to stay healthy. I remember going to the local "*Vaidya*" (Ayurvedic physician) or homeopath for minor ailments to help us recover faster. Due to our preventive lifestyle, we hardly used to fall sick or have fevers in early childhood. We were a family of larks (early risers), typically waking up at 5 am or so, all bright-eyed and cheerful, and then as kids, we used to be in bed and fast asleep by 9 pm.

I remember being extremely open to integrative modalities and tools during my medical school training in India. For example, I recommended probiotics routinely to patients if they were prescribed antibiotics for any reason. I also started my intensive yoga training and practiced during my first year of medical college and studied the Homeopathic Materia Medica during those years. Maintaining my good health—despite the stress and time pressures of medical college—was easy as I followed a health-supportive lifestyle.

I was in peak health until I came to the USA for my medical residency. During the challenging four years of training, working an average of 36 hours in a shift, living in a stressful urban-city environment in New York, with total dissociation from the natural intelligence of nature and its rhythmic cycles, away from the proximity of my family and loved ones and my strong nurturing social support system, I noticed a gradual decline in my health.

Since I was new to the USA, I was not aware that the cold northeast with short summers and spending all our waking hours inside the hospital had caused me to develop Vitamin D deficiency and made my moods fluctuate. Nor was I aware that the easy shortcut, microwave cooking was not the ideal way of cooking, or that the highly stressful charged environment in the hospital, taking care of critically sick patients for prolonged hours and significant sleep deprivation, was draining my adrenal reserve.

The underlying issues festered and climaxed after a few years of (unknowingly) eating GMO foods. These foods were highly sprayed with glyphosate, the perfect setup for leaky gut, which led to autoimmune issues, skin breakouts, joint aches/pain, and dysfunctional gut symptoms. Despite my busy schedule, I tried to regain some degree of health by continuing to practice my yoga, pranayama, and meditation techniques intermittently. But it was an ongoing challenge.

Now trained in the standard Western model and expected to keep functioning in that fast-paced role, I felt I lacked the proper skill set to heal people. I was tired of offering "Band-Aid" therapies that temporarily mitigate symptoms but then cause more side effects. We were not taught to look at the root cause of disease. I remember a patient asking me about the side effects of an inactive ingredient of her prescribed medication and asking for natural alternatives. I was frozen at that moment as I did not feel confident offering her any lifestyle or integrative options due to cultural differences.

New to the practice of medicine in the USA, I was brainwashed into believing that a new medicine for diabetes mellitus was "a revolutionary medicine in the last several decades." I remember the trauma and guilt when further safety studies led to the medication being recalled five years later. I called many patients for whom I had prescribed that medicine and reviewed the safety data with them before switching their medications. The guilt weighed heavily on my heart. It took years and hard work to release its grip on me. And my professional dissatisfaction kept growing.

Soon after, I got married and decided to take a sabbatical. After receiving encouragement from my husband, I went back to India to train extensively in the ancient healing science and art of <u>Ayurveda</u>, <u>Acupuncture</u>, advanced <u>Yoga</u> training, and various <u>meditation</u> practices, including <u>SKY Breath</u> from Art of Living and <u>Vipassana</u> technique.

When I returned to the USA, I felt better equipped to take on the challenges of truly healing the world. I was also determined to regain the vitality and vibrant health I had until my early adult years. So, I decided to further educate myself in <u>Functional Medicine</u>, <u>Integrative Medicine</u>, and <u>Lifestyle Medicine,</u> among other advanced training and certifications, like mindfulness from the Center for Mind-Body Medicine <u>(CMBM)</u>, <u>Biofeedback</u>, traditional yogic practices like <u>Isha Yoga</u>, etc. to expand my toolbox with healing modalities. Then, I could offer my patients the best comprehensive skill set and healing tools.

Deciding to turn my life around, I practiced meditation and yoga regularly. I learned that I was sensitive to gluten and gave it up completely. I also became a vegan. I had been a whole food plant-based (WFPB) vegetarian since childhood and previously experimented with being a pescatarian. I cleaned up my diet, favoring local, seasonal, and organic foods from the farmers market, and started cooking three fresh meals daily. I started practicing mindful eating and let go of my medical school/residency ingrained habit of swallowing my meals over 2–3 minutes. I intentionally created time to tend my organic garden after work and used to come back late in the evening, totally refreshed and filled with energy. We grew rows of strawberries, raspberries, various fruit trees, seasonal herbs and veggies, and meadows of colorful wildflowers in our garden. I spend hours in the acreages after work, playing in the soil, just rejuvenating and relaxing, watching the butterflies and bees buzzing at work incessantly, the frogs croak in the gentle creek with the mild pitter-patter of rain, the deer and fawns rest in shade, the wild birds flock to the feeders in falling snow, and the wild turkeys dance across our lawns.

This filled me with a sense of awe and wonder at the beauty and generosity of mother earth and filled my heart with gratitude for all the abundance nature has provided us to help not just our physical but also mental, emotional, and spiritual well-being. I discovered the power of *Gratitude* and noticed a major shift in my heart, opening energetically and gradually refilling with kindness and compassion for all beings [2].

Benefits of Exposure to Nature

Evidence suggests nature's role in improving multiple aspects of human health, ranging from pre-birth to elderly, including:

- Reduction of stress, anxiety, depression, and improved attention deficit disorders.
- Increased positive affect, well-being, and increased incidence of good self-reported health.
- Improved sleep, cognition, and feeling rested.
- Reductions in diastolic blood pressure, heart rate, and Improved heart rate variability (HRV)
- Decreased incidence of diabetes, dyslipidemia, asthma, obesity, and cardiovascular diseases.
- Decreased preterm births and low birth weights.
- Decreased all-cause, stroke-specific, and CVD mortality.
- Improved physical activity and pain control.
- Boosting immune system functioning and decreased salivary cortisol (stress marker).
- Decreased Incidences of urban crimes.
- Reduction in exposure to air pollutants, noise and excessive heat.
- Increased social connectedness and regard for the environment. [3,4]

Nature as Medicine: Did you know?

- Exposure to Nature supports multiple health benefits spanning physical, mental, emotional, cognitive, social, and biophysiological domains. [5]
- Green space (any space containing vegetation and associated with natural elements, for example, parks, urban forests, playgrounds, tree-lined streets, riverbanks etc.) can influence our planetary health. [6]
- The World Health Organization recommends that all people reside within 300m of green space. Within cities, the degree of greening varies across neighborhoods, with less and lower quality green space typically found in communities of lower socio-economic status. [7]
- Many ancestral traditions and civilizations, including ancient Egyptians, Chinese, Persians, Indians, and First Nation and indigenous peoples around the world have considered Nature as healing. [8]
- Biophilia ("love of life") describes the human drive to connect with nature and other living things. [9] Harvard Biologist Edward O. Wilson proposed that humans' attraction to nature is genetically predetermined and the result of evolution in his 1984 book 'Biophilia.' [10]
- The Japanese Ministry of Agriculture, Forestry, and Fisheries coined the term 'shinrin-yoku' or forest-bathing in 1982. Time spent in nature has been associated with increased expression of anti-cancer proteins and natural killer (NK) cells— immune cells that can kill tumor cells or cells infected with viruses. [11]
- Trees and plants emit 'phytoncides', essential oils that protect flora from parasites and germs. When we breathe in these natural antimicrobials, they increase natural killer cell activity, promote higher immunity, and work as anti-inflammatories that reduce oxidative stress, enhance sleep via alpha-pinene, reduce cortisol levels, and reduce blood glucose levels. [12]

It has been an arduous journey of self-healing for me. This self-healing typically comes late to most physicians as we always offer to heal others, pushing through our own health battles and always helping others, even though our cups might be empty. Slowly but surely, I overcame most of my medical issues, gradually reclaiming my health and thriving again with energy.

Over the last two decades, the worsening and decline of the Western healthcare model have come to the forefront. The COVID-19 pandemic brought to prominence the shortcomings of the system and rampant burnout of healthcare providers (HCP). I have personally been through several cycles of near-burnout to complete burnout in the last decade due to the changing environment, increasing workload due to high HCP turnover rates, lack of control and autonomy, increased administrative burden, lack of support, and increased pressure from administrative staff to see more patients and increase "numbers," which are publicly compared in meetings to shame the "poor performers," the HCP.

The stress of daily life in medicine can be overwhelming, making it especially applicable for HCP to utilize the stress management pillar of LM. The WHO describes burnout as defined in the 11th Revision of the International Classification of Diseases (ICD-11) as "resulting from chronic workplace stress that has not been successfully managed," characterized by "feelings of energy depletion or exhaustion, increased mental distance from one's job, or feelings of negativism or cynicism related to one's job; and reduced professional efficacy" [13]. Early research on burnout showed it to be a fundamentally systemic problem. More recent researchers also describe the causes of burnout as collective and impossible for an individual to fix without a systems perspective.

We must recognize that it is not just our personal resilience that can save us from these cycles of burnout but also much-needed organizational changes that need to happen. We must be motivated and guided toward increasing health behaviors and reconnecting to a greater sense of meaning and purpose, enhancing professional fulfillment, preventing burnout, and living a more connected life.

It is time for us, as true healers, to take back healing into our own hands again, away from the business-oriented system riddled with middle management whose only priority is to bring more dollars to the table, regardless of whether it is at the cost of the health of HCPs, physicians, or patients. The current monetary-based system has seemingly lost its "soul and purpose" of healing, and we need to stand united in our efforts to regain it back for the benefit of all of our patients and us.

Fortunately, the last few years have led to growing awareness of the inadequacy of the system, both for healthcare workers who are struggling with burnout or looking to address the root cause of disease for patients. Instead of putting "patchwork Band-Aids," there's a shifting focus on treating the cause of erupting lifestyle-related chronic, non-communicable diseases—most of which are preventable as we know now. Staying open to and learning more evidence-based healing tools such as Lifestyle Medicine tools, Integrative Medicine modalities, and Mind-Body Medicine techniques helps empower clinicians to help their patients and their community.

The medicine paradigm is shifting from primarily physically focused treatment to encompassing the bio-psych-social approach to health. This comprehensive model is proactive, preventative, patient-centered, and addresses the whole person. There is strong evolving evidence on the importance of following the six pillars of LM, including a whole food plant-predominant eating pattern, physical activity, restorative sleep, stress management, avoidance of risky substances, and nurturing positive social connections and relationships. Upcoming evidence in the emerging field of positive psychology encourages us to use many of these interventions to improve our own and the population's health. Health professionals, who learn techniques to maintain and improve their physical and emotional well-being, manage their stress levels, and flourish, will be better equipped to educate and empower their patients too.

A lifestyle medicine approach to population care has the potential to arrest and reverse the decades-long explosion of chronic conditions and their burdensome healthcare and personal cost. Patient and provider satisfaction increases from a LM approach. It strongly aligns the LM field with the Quintuple Aim of better health outcomes, lower cost, improved patient satisfaction, improved provider well-being, and advancement of health equity, in addition to its alignment with planetary health [14].

I continue to be amazed at the unlimited wisdom of our ancient seers, yogis, and scientists, who excelled in the science of yoga and Āyurveda thousands of years ago. The modern evidence being unraveled about the mind-body connection, relaxation response, biofeedback, autogenics, clinical hypnosis, gut-brain connection, the microbiome, circadian rhythm, sleep cycles, biofield energy, the power of breathwork, heart rate variability, gratitude, compassion, and more, had their roots and origin in these ancient wise cultures. The evolving science of happiness and positive psychology has many lessons to be learned from the ancient sciences of yoga, Ayurveda, and other traditional wisdom, including the philosophy of *Ahimsa* (non-violence at all levels), *Asteya* (non-coveting), *Santosha* (contentment), and *Satya* (truthfulness).

I continue to work on walking this path toward unraveling my life's authentic and higher purpose and guiding and supporting others to achieve their life goals too. My life lessons and journey, thus far, have inspired me to dedicate my knowledge—spanning from ancient healing wisdom pearls to the latest evidence-based lifestyle, functional and integrative medicine recommendations—to my patients and my community and offer an intuitive, compassionate approach to unravel our body's innate ability to heal. I have worked with thousands of patients in my practice, guiding and coaching them to find clues and answers deep within themselves and utilizing the skill sets I taught them. Their personal transformations to living a life full of joy, hope, love, abundance, vibrant health, and synchronous living with the intelligence of nature are remarkable. Not only have my patients and I benefited, but also my family, friends, and social connections have been impacted favorably by my being more present, and sharing beautiful times together, allowing us to create wonderful memories.

"Make your life a journey of service."
— Dr. Prachi Garodia

What does having Meaning and Purpose in Life mean?

Our sense of Meaning and purpose in life are very personal, subjective and can change through our life's journey. Meaning is how we "make sense of life and our roles in it," Purpose is the "aspirations that motivate our activities." [15]

In his book, Man's Search for Meaning [16], Victor Frankl described meaning as a principal human need, allowing self-transcendence (an ability to develop a purpose beyond the self). He stated that meaning could be found in three ways:
- through work and creative efforts,
- through relationships, and
- through the attitude we take (or reappraisals we make) toward unavoidable suffering.

I invite you to dedicate some self-care time to meditate and contemplate on your own Life's meaning and Purpose.

You deserve it!!

This chapter is dedicated to my ever-loving parents, my siblings, and my supportive husband, who have all been my cheerleaders in this life's journey.

References:

1. White, N., Bautista, V., Lenz, T., & Cosimano, A. (2020). Using the SMART-EST Goals in Lifestyle Medicine Prescription. *American Journal of Lifestyle Medicine, 14*(3), 271–273. https://doi.org/10.1177/1559827620905775

2. Millacci, T. S., PhD. (2023). What is Gratitude and Why Is It So Important? *PositivePsychology.com.* https://positivepsychology.com/gratitude-appreciation/

3. Victorson, D., Luberto, C. M., & Koffler, K. (2020). Nature As Medicine: Mind, Body, and Soil. *The Journal of Alternative and Complementary Medicine, 26*(8), 658–662. https://doi.org/10.1089/acm.2020.0221

4. Twohig-Bennett, C., & Jones, A. (2018). The health benefits of the great outdoors: A systematic review and meta-analysis of greenspace exposure and health outcomes. *Environmental Research, 166*, 628–637. https://doi.org/10.1016/j.envres.2018.06.030

5. Seymour, V. (2016). The Human–Nature Relationship and its Impact on Health: A Critical review. *Frontiers in Public Health, 4.* https://doi.org/10.3389/fpubh.2016.00260

6. Sobstyl, J. M., Emig, T., Qomi, M. J. A., Ulm, F., & Pellenq, R. J. (2018). Role of city texture in urban heat islands at nighttime. *Physical Review Letters, 120*(10). https://doi.org/10.1103/physrevlett.120.108701

7. World Health Organization. Regional Office for Europe. (2016). *Urban green spaces and health.* https://apps.who.int/iris/handle/10665/345751

8. Coates, P. (2013). *Nature: Western Attitudes Since Ancient*

Times. John Wiley & Sons.

9. Kellert, S. R., & Wilson, E. O. (1995). *The Biophilia Hypothesis*. Island Press.

10. Wilson, E. O. (2009). *Biophilia*. https://doi.org/10.2307/j.ctv k12s6h

11. Li, Q., Morimoto, K., Nakadai, A., Inagaki, H., Katsumata, M., Shimizu, T., Hirata, Y., Hirata, K., Suzuki, H., Miyazaki, Y., Kagawa, T., Koyama, Y., Ohira, T., Takayama, N., Krensky, A. M., & Kawada, T. (2007). Forest bathing enhances human natural killer activity and expression of Anti-Cancer proteins. *International Journal of Immunopathology and Pharmacology*, *20*(2_suppl), 3–8. https://doi.org/10.1177/03946320070200 s202

12. Antonelli, M., Donelli, D., Barbieri, G., Valussi, M., Maggini, V., & Firenzuoli, F. (2020). Forest volatile Organic Compounds and their Effects on Human Health: A State-of-the-Art Review. *International Journal of Environmental Research and Public Health*, *17*(18), 6506. https://doi.org/10.3390/ijerph171865 06

13. World Health Organization: WHO. (2019, May 28). Burn-out an "occupational phenomenon": International Classification of Diseases. *WHO*. https://www.who.int/news/item/28-05-2019-burn-out-an-oc cupational-phenomenon-international-classification-of-diseas es

14. Nundy, S., Cooper, L. A., & Mate, K. S. (2022). The Quintuple Aim for Health Care Improvement. *JAMA*, *327*(6), 521. http s://doi.org/10.1001/jama.2021.25181

15. Ivtzan, I., Young, T., Martman, J., Jeffrey, A., Lomas, T.,

Hart, R., & Eiroa-Orosa, F. J. (2016). Integrating Mindfulness into Positive Psychology: a Randomised Controlled Trial of an Online Positive Mindfulness Program. *Mindfulness*, *7*(6), 1396–1407. https://doi.org/10.1007/s12671-016-0581-1

16. Frankl, V. E. (1946). *Man's search for meaning.* http://lifemanagement4filipinos.weebly.com/uploads/1/2/0/6/12062185/mans search for meaning - viktor e. frankl 1.pdf

About Dr. Prachi Garodia, MD, ABIM, ABIHM, DipABLM, DipAyu, NBC-HWC

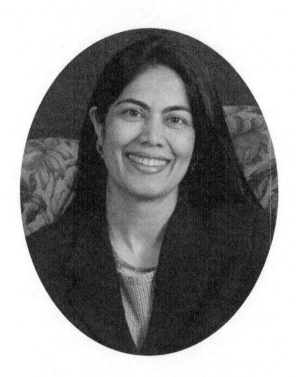

Dr. Prachi Garodia is board certified in Internal Medicine, a board-certified Diplomate in Integrative Medicine and Lifestyle Medicine, and a nationally board-certified Health and Wellness Coach. She has also trained in Functional Medicine, Ayurveda, Yoga, Acupuncture (Medical, Cosmetic, and Electro-Acupuncture), Meditation, Mindfulness techniques, Positive Psychology, Biofeedback, and Clinical Hypnosis, among other modalities.

Dr. Garodia is a certified instructor of Battlefield acupuncture at the Veterans Health Administration (VHA), a certified trainer for Mind-Body Medicine through the CMBM, an iRest Yoga Nidra Level 2 Trainer, a certified Heartmath Resilience Advantage Trainer, a yoga instructor, and faculty at VaYU for M.Sc. in Yoga Therapy. Dr. Garodia is helping create a new course on Mantram meditation at the VHA, training to become a Tai Chi facilitator, and pursuing a master's and trainer certification in Aromatherapy. She embodies a child-like playfulness, curiosity, and a growth mindset and is passionate about helping her healthcare colleagues learn to heal by utilizing their body's innate healing ability.

Dr. Garodia currently serves as the National Education Champion for Whole Health through the Office of Patient-Centered Care and Cultural Transformation (OPCC&CT) at the VHA, as Clinical Director and Section Chief for Whole Health at Miami Veterans Affairs (VA) facility, as the co-chair of the happiness science and positive health Member Interest Group (MIG) of the American College of Lifestyle Medicine (ACLM) for 2021–2024, a member for happiness science and positive health committee for ACLM, and on the Board for Global Positive Health Institute. In addition, Dr. Garodia has served as a medical director for VA ECHO VISN 20 Education and on the board of directors for several nonprofits over the years.

Dr. Garodia has published several journal articles related to inflammation, chronic diseases, and cancer, co-authored a chapter for an Ayurvedic reference book, and is working on several articles, book chapters, and her own book.

Dr. Garodia is an empathic healer, Ayurvedic chef, master gardener, environmentalist, and a whole foods plant-based advocate. Her journey in Integrative Medicine started 25+ years ago with her training in the ancient science of Ayurveda, yoga, and meditation. She has been educating, learning, and growing with her colleagues and patients since then.

Dr. Garodia is an avid master gardener and practices yoga and meditation, dancing with abandon with friends, traveling, spending time in nature, camping, and hiking with her husband. In addition, she is a health foodie and finds joy in creating delicious and easy plant-based recipes for her friends and family. For her, "Food IS Medicine" and "Nature Is the Best Healer." Her patients have nicknamed her "The Healing MD."

For more information, please check out the following:

Website: https://www.drprachigarodia.com/

and http://www.thehealingmdllc.com/

Facebook: https://www.facebook.com/drgarodia/

Instagram: https://www.instagram.com/the_healing_md/

LinkedIn: https://www.linkedin.com/in/prachi-garodia-md-8947921
09/

Twitter: https://twitter.com/prachigarodiamd

Watch an interview with the co-author:

6

From Surviving to Living, a Journey

Sirisha Guthikonda, MD, DipABLM

"The greatest wealth is health."

— Virgil

During my adolescence, I achieved an active life naturally. I loved playing various sports and eating home-cooked meals. Both aspects paused in my life as I entered medical school. The long and late studying hours interfered with my athleticism. Getting my meals from outside my home became the new norm. This continued into my post-training life. My health post-pregnancy revealed the consequence of these decisions, which had built up over the years. Around the same time, my husband's cholesterol was 4–5 times higher than normal, a severely elevated level that opened my eyes to our current lifestyle. Realizing the path we were taking with our everyday choices, I decided to start making changes at home.

I found videos of an Indian naturopath who helped many people with his plant-based diet. A close relative of mine had followed his strict diet plan and lost 30 pounds. She was able to decrease her diabetes and blood pressure medications. Inspired by this knowledge and other success stories, I made changes in how I prepared food, started eating more plant-based meals, and ate at home as much as possible. However, I still required medication for my thyroid disease and persistent fatigue. Around the same time, my family asked me about the keto diet. Initially, the keto diet started as a possible intriguing answer to our health challenges. After reading about it, we decided to try it. We all tried the keto diet together, and we were able to lose considerable weight. Given its restrictive nature, the keto diet didn't seem to be sustainable for us. We soon stopped the diet, and we all gained back the weight.

Frustrated with this fluctuating weight, I decided not to go on any other diet but rather make one small change at a time, which is more practical given our busy lifestyle. The hardest part of this whole process was avoiding sweets altogether. You see, I have a bit of a sweet tooth! I noticed the more I tried to avoid sweets, the more I wanted to eat them. I found a balance by having a small portion of sweets after lunch. I noticed I had more energy after making these diet changes and incorporating regular exercise into my routine at least four days a week. I was also able to get off my thyroid medication! I began sharing these lifestyle changes with my family, close friends, and patients.

I inspired one of my patients, who was overweight and struggling with arthritis. She went off of all sugars and processed food. It resulted in a 20-pound weight loss and improvement in her blood pressure and cholesterol numbers. Furthermore, due to her weight loss, she was finally able to undergo successful hip replacement with a rapid recovery after surgery.

While I was passionate about helping people, I felt stuck after a certain point in my career and knew I could do more than just my formal Nephrology (specialty of kidneys) practice. After consulting a friend about possible ways to initiate sustainable change, she mentioned an interesting field called Lifestyle Medicine (LM), in which she had a study group going. I joined the group and learned about the six fundamental pillars behind LM. Learning about the possibilities of relieving and even reversing diseases with implementable lifestyle changes was exciting. I was convinced this was a true game changer and eventually completed the board certification for LM.

After the certification, I realized one of the biggest risk factors for cardiovascular disease is inactivity, more than smoking. I always loved outdoor activities and sports, but with work and family commitments, exercise went down to the bottom of the list and was neglected over the years. To combat this problem, I started walking and yoga, which were the best decisions I made for my physical health. After practicing for several months, I noticed how my strength and energy levels were significantly better.

I began my solo medical practice not too long after completing my LM board certification and started to educate my patients about the six pillars of LM. I hoped to inspire them about lifestyle medicine, just as the field has done for me. I could see the differences in the lab results of my patients after they started implementing lifestyle changes. I remember one patient, in particular, undergoing chemotherapy and struggling with obesity, diabetes, high blood pressure, and lack of energy. After discussing this with me, she made the necessary lifestyle changes, including minimizing red meats, adding regular exercise, and sleeping better. Her health radically improved. She lost weight and improved her high blood pressure, diabetes, and kidney function. Overall, she had more energy, even on chemotherapy.

Another impressive transformation I have seen was in a patient with high blood pressure, kidney disease, and lupus who also cut down on red meats, and processed foods, and increased veggies after counseling with me. With the help of lifestyle changes, not only did she see an improvement in her blood pressure but also a great improvement in her kidney function and inflammatory markers. I have noticed this improvement in many of my patients. As they started to minimize red meats, avoid processed foods, and eat a more plant-based diet, not only has their kidney function improved, but so has their blood pressure, overall energy levels, and metabolic health.

Initially, I thought it would be easy to lead a better life after being thoroughly educated on the benefits of these practices. However, I quickly came to realize it was not so simple. With the culture of long working hours, easy availability of processed food, and the pricey options of healthy foods, improving one's lifestyle takes much more than just knowing the right things to do.

With this realization came the struggles of practical implementation. I have recently experienced this when I had difficulty finding healthy food options at local events such as theme parks or carnivals. I ended up eating pizza, feeling frustrated both by the lack of options and frustrated that I had not been prepared by bringing backup food with me.

Other challenges include the food served in the school cafeterias. My daughter naturally wanted to buy the school lunch like her friends. The school lunch menu mostly had processed food, which was disheartening. Most kids get used to these addictive fried foods at such an early age. It becomes hard to change their habits to health-conscious ones. Today's kids are the pillars of our future but are living on a suboptimal diet. I believe if we teach kids about nutrition and the importance of lifestyle at an early age, not only does it become easier for them to follow when they grow up, but also it will also help avoid the metabolic disease pandemic we are facing now.

I have learned that it is not about being perfect all the time but about starting with one small, doable change at a time. Starting with only one habit, such as getting enough water daily, can be a goal to focus on until it has become a habit. After it has become second nature, start practicing and applying the next habit that becomes the main focus, and only then can healthy choices be built and sustained over time. Like a ladder, take one step at a time.

Since my family has started this journey of implementing the teachings of lifestyle medicine into our home, my husband's cholesterol level has normalized with a combination of medication and lifestyle changes. With additional dietary changes and exercise, his medication dose decreased. We have a ways to go, but we do realize it's a process and takes conscious effort. This can only be achieved if we understand the "why" behind our actions. We still go out to eat and eat what is available at social gatherings, albeit more consciously and intentionally than before. It is important to relax and enjoy the events and company of family and friends. Our mental well-being and social connections are just as important, and these gatherings help boost it.

Throughout this process, I have learned an incredible amount about the impact of a proper lifestyle on one's overall health. Despite not being taught this when I was in medical school, it is exciting to see that lifestyle medicine is being incorporated into more recent residency programs. I am hopeful that one day we will see more importance given to preventative medicine. As the saying goes, "Prevention is the best medicine."

Dedicated to my family, who have been supportive throughout my journey.

About Dr. Sirisha Guthikonda, MD, DipABLM

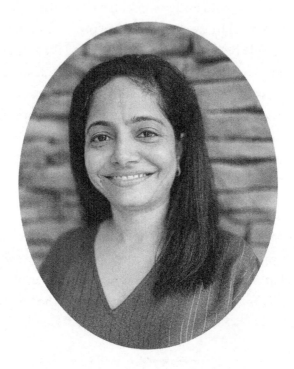

Dr. Sirisha Guthikonda is a practicing Nephrologist in Atlanta, Georgia, USA. She is triple board certified in Internal Medicine, Nephrology, and Lifestyle Medicine. She is passionate about empowering patients through education, helping them understand the underlying problem, and adopting a sustainable healthy lifestyle change. She also volunteers in free local clinics. In her leisure time, she enjoys yoga, hiking, cooking, and spending time with family and friends.

Watch an interview with the co-author:

DR. SIRISHA
GUTHIKONDA

Scan Me

7

FRACTURED TO HEALED: A PHYSICIAN'S PERSONAL EXPERIENCE WITH LIFESTYLE MEDICINE

Kelley Hagerich, MD, MPH, FACP, DipABOM, DipABLM

"The wound is the place where the light enters you."

— Rumi

The Cardiology attending physician was hustling around in a flurry of activity in hopes of saving our patient's life. I was on my cardiac ICU rotation during my internal medicine residency in Pittsburgh, near where I grew up in rural Pennsylvania. This young man, not yet even thirty years old and close to my age, was spiraling into worsening heart failure that was unlikely to be adequately treated with medications alone. The several hundred extra pounds he had put on in his twenties caused him to develop obesity-induced heart failure. The only viable treatment option for him by this time was a heart transplant. Unfortunately, his weight disqualified him from being a transplant candidate. His situation was heartbreaking for not only the patient and his family but also the medical staff. The Cardiology attending physician made phone call after phone call to try and get the young man urgent gastric bypass surgery so that he could lose weight as quickly as possible and, thus, get on the list for a heart transplant. But we all knew in our hearts that bariatric surgery would be high-risk for him and would not be performed on an urgent basis. I rotated to a different medical service shortly thereafter. I never knew what happened to this young man, but his story left an impression on me and my future career path.

During my internal medicine residency, I came to realize that the reflexive nature of prescribing medications to treat patients' established medical problems did not fit with my personal philosophy of how I wanted to practice medicine. I wanted to hear about patients' lives, their families, their interests, and how their paths through the world influenced their health, but there was little time to really talk to patients. I became increasingly unhappy in my training, but I was not aware of how to challenge and change the status quo. Despite my discontent, I pushed myself to complete residency while neglecting my own health and well-being. I ate whatever food was available to me in the hospital, no matter how unhealthy, exercised infrequently, and considered regular sleep a luxury. My stress level was constantly high, and I neglected my personal relationships with family and friends. The only healthy behavior I practiced was avoiding unhealthy substance use.

When H1N1 influenza went tearing through the population of Pittsburgh during the third and last year of my residency, I should not have been surprised that my unhealthy behaviors set me up to become seriously ill after I became infected. I was hospitalized for several days and out of work for weeks. When I was able to return to work, I was short of breath while rounding on patients in the hospital and battled crushing fatigue, but I still pushed myself onward. Following this illness with H1N1 influenza, I developed a series of medical problems within the last few months of my training. I noticed while running around the hospital that I could not lift or flex my left foot. As I quickly walked down a long hallway to a patient's hospital room, the only thing I heard was the sound of my left foot slapping against the ground. I recognized this condition as foot drop, which usually presents in neurologic conditions, such as multiple sclerosis. I was overcome with fear, but I knew this symptom could not be ignored. I saw a physician colleague who arranged for neurological testing with an EMG, which showed nerve damage to my peroneal nerve. The testing suggested that the pressure in the muscle compartments in my lower legs was too high. I underwent pressure testing by having a large needle inserted into my leg while I walked on a treadmill, which was painful, to say the least.

I was diagnosed with exertional compartment syndrome in both my legs, although it was far worse in my left leg, which had progressed to the point of causing nerve damage. Similar to how I felt crushed in my professional life, the muscles in my leg were compressing the nerves and vasculature, causing pain and nerve damage. The orthopedic surgeon I saw recommended surgery within the next few weeks to cut open the fascia of my lower leg compartments and relieve the pressure. In the last month of my residency, I had unexpected surgery on both of my lower legs at the same time. I hobbled to my residency graduation dinner on crutches with heavily swollen legs and in significant pain. It took the loss of my ability to walk on my own to realize that I was at a personal and professional crossroads. All I knew at this point was that I needed a different approach to my own health and my practice of medicine. I wanted to prevent my patients from developing health problems in the first place. If I could prevent disease, I could prevent suffering. I realized that I needed to start with myself.

Following completion of my internal medicine residency training, I moved across the country to San Diego to start a second residency in General Preventive Medicine and Public Health. I viewed my move to San Diego as a fresh start for my career and for my health. My excitement to learn more about not just disease but also health, well-being, and prevention could barely be contained. For my own health, I started physical therapy to gain back the strength and functioning of my legs after my unexpected surgery shortly before my move. I also started working with a nutritionist and explored nutrition on my own by reading books and exploring healthy grocery store options. However, my stress level remained high, my sleep quality was poor, and I found it difficult to get my personal relationships back on track after neglecting them for three years during my internal medicine residency. Unfortunately, despite my initial efforts to improve my health, it continued to decline. I developed recurrent infections, including sinusitis, bronchitis, and conjunctivitis. Pretty much every "-itis" that comes to mind. I flew back to Pennsylvania for the holidays to visit with my family, but within 24 hours of arriving, I found myself hospitalized with a severe case of gastroenteritis. I spent Christmas Day in the hospital, which was not how I planned to spend my limited vacation time.

I started to have a niggling thought in the back of my head that there was something seriously wrong with my immune system. After seeing two immunologists, my initial suspicion regarding my immune system proved correct. I was diagnosed with a rare primary immunodeficiency called common variable immunodeficiency (CVID). It was a condition that I barely remembered learning about during medical school and had only seen once during my residency. With this disease, my body does not make enough functioning antibodies to protect me against infection. CVID also means that many routine vaccines do not work in these patients like me. The treatment for CVID is lifelong immunoglobulin (IgG) replacement therapy made from plasma pooled from thousands of donors. I elected to administer my IgG therapy at home subcutaneously on a weekly basis. It was difficult to accept being a patient while I continued to work as a physician. I felt like a failure because my efforts to improve my own health had not been successful. There I was at 29 years old, now committed to a lifetime of worrying not only about my risk of infection but also about how to maintain continuous health insurance to pay for my prohibitively expensive IgG therapy.

When I graduated from my preventive medicine residency in 2012, the field of Lifestyle Medicine (LM) was in its infancy and was initially a small offshoot of the field of preventive medicine. Originally, I had hoped to enter a preventive medicine career in public health, such as the

Epidemic Intelligence Service with the CDC. However, my diagnosis of CVID derailed my career plans and life plans. My condition felt like a ball and chain, keeping me in one location to allow me to continue my regular IgG treatments. I quickly came to realize that after graduating from my preventive medicine residency, I needed a steady job with good health insurance and minimal travel. My immunologist gave me the approval to return to clinical medicine with some precautions. I applied and was offered a job in the Primary Care Department at the local hospital. I stayed in this job for the next nine years, barely treading water in my career and personal life. While I was able to negotiate limited time to work in the obesity clinic, I was otherwise entirely consumed by the needs of my primary care patients and the never-ending paperwork and responsibilities of that job.

With each passing year, my workload continued to grow to an unsustainable amount. I was working from home for hours in the evening and on the weekends just to keep afloat. My discontent with my career deepened, and my physical health continued to worsen. My diet was poor and unbalanced. I began treating myself to M&Ms from the vending machine at work just to get through the day. The weight piled on, but I barely noticed. I needed a sleeping pill to get to sleep at night, and I still felt fatigued all the time. It was easy to attribute my malaise and unhappiness as a by-product of my CVID. I had given up on taking care of myself because I felt that my previous efforts had not prevented me from developing CVID. However irrational it was, I told myself there was no point in trying to feel better now when doing so would not cure my disease.

When the COVID-19 pandemic made its appearance in March 2020, I left my office on a Friday afternoon and knew that I did not feel safe returning to the office the following Monday. I did not know that I would never return to my office again. While my IgG therapy protected me against most known infections, COVID was an entirely different beast. My IgG therapy takes at least a year to make from donated plasma. This lag time in production meant it would be a minimum of a year until

I could even consider that there would be any protection against COVID in my IgG therapy. I was granted a reasonable accommodation from my job to see my patients via telemedicine from home. I lived alone with my dog and found myself entering what turned out to be a year of complete physical isolation.

While I was thankful to be safely sequestered at home and still working, I found myself growing increasingly restless. I tried to spend as much time as I could outside. In December 2020, I broke my foot jumping out of the way of a speeding car while walking my dog. Unfortunately, it turned out to be a fifth metatarsal fracture, which is known for being difficult to heal. I saw a podiatrist and an orthopedic surgeon. I had numerous X-rays and an MRI. I wore a walking boot and used a knee scooter for months. Despite these efforts and time, there was no healing of my fracture. I then tried using a bone stimulator for several months without relief. Amid all this chaos with my foot, I continued practicing primary care via telemedicine from home since it was exceedingly difficult for me to get around. I did not realize that things were about to get even worse for me.

One afternoon in March 2021, I went into my bedroom to get something and noticed an inch of steaming water covering my bedroom floor. It turned out that the hot water heater in the adjoining room had malfunctioned and had leaked through my bedroom wall. All my belongings on the floor of my bedroom were destroyed and had to be thrown away. In addition, the walls and floor of my bedroom had to be ripped out and replaced to prevent the growth of mold. I had to move out and into a hotel for two weeks while my home was repaired and made livable again. I could not imagine a more medically stressful time for myself. I had a broken foot and had to use a knee scooter to get around in a hotel. Also, while I had had my first dose of the COVID-19 vaccine at this point, no one could say whether the vaccine would be effective in patients like me who were immunosuppressed.

As I sat alone in my bland hotel room, trying to see my own primary care patients via video, I had an epiphany. I realized how unhappy I was in my personal and professional life, and I had reached my breaking point. Working in primary care felt like a never-ending stream of appointments in which I was prescribing the same medications over and over to treat the same handful of conditions. Most of the conditions I treated were related to lifestyle and were preventable, such as diabetes mellitus, hypertension, and hyperlipidemia. It was frustrating that I did not have the time or the support in my job to adequately treat the root causes of these diseases by addressing my patients' lifestyle choices. I knew I could not continue in this position for another nine years or even another year. I had been threatening for years to get a new job, but I had not put forth a concerted effort primarily because I was so worn out from surviving the day-to-day grind of my job.

In addition, besides my CVID and my nonunion foot fracture, my overall state of health was poor. I was overweight, physically inactive, eating a low-quality diet, depressed, anxious, and stressed, and had poor, fragmented sleep. I felt isolated with limited daily social support since it was difficult to meet up with friends because of my medical conditions. As I cleaned out my ruined belongings from my flooded bedroom, wheeling back and forth on my knee scooter to the outdoor trash can, I realized it was time to let go. The flood, while stressful at the time, served a purpose for me. It showed me that I needed to clear out the physical and mental clutter from my life to focus on what was truly important to me. I knew as I threw away my half-used journals, forgotten books, soggy clothing, shoes, and ruined furniture, that while I was attached to these things in that moment of time, I would not even remember them in the future. I realized it was time to change my life, and the changes had to start from within myself.

I decided that I would completely change my life over the next year. In one year, I hoped to be in a much better place physically, emotionally, and mentally. It took a few months to gather my activation energy to start my transformation, but once I started one change, I hoped that one positive change would snowball into other positive changes. I realized that I needed to change my job before I could make meaningful changes to the rest of my life. At that time, I was spending all my free time working, and I felt physically and emotionally depleted at the end of each day. I began identifying small, concrete changes in my life that I could make. I started networking over the summer of 2021, and I learned of a full-time job in obesity medicine with a focus on lifestyle medicine at another healthcare facility. Within a few weeks of learning about the job, I applied, interviewed, and was offered my dream job. I gave several months' notice to my first job and started my new job in obesity medicine in January 2022.

Soon after submitting my resignation to the job I had held for nine years, I felt tremendous relief and overall lighter. Once I had a plan in place for my career, I felt that I could devote more time and energy to improving my health. I decided to start my life makeover by working on my sleep. I had not slept well in years and had issues with both falling asleep and staying asleep. I started wearing a sleep-tracking ring at night that gave me insight and recommendations on how to improve my sleep. I read articles and books about sleep. I limited my screen time and wore blue-light-blocking glasses. Gradually, my sleep started to improve incrementally, and the pervasive fatigue hanging over me slowly started to lift. I also began overhauling my diet and worked on learning to cook healthy plant-based meals. As the flood had cleaned out the clutter in my life, I decided I needed to clean out other unhealthy corners of my life. I started in the kitchen by throwing away unhealthy food and began accumulating a healthier supply of food. I tried different meal prep kits and cooked for myself more.

I invested in bettering myself by changing my lifestyle. I began identifying as a healthy person and made choices that aligned with that identity. When I returned to see my orthopedic surgeon in March 2022, I had a positive feeling that things would be better. Together, we looked at the newest X-ray of my foot, zooming in and looking at it from multiple angles. There was no sign of a fracture. We could not even see any evidence of where the fracture had been. In the intervening months since I had last seen my orthopedic surgeon, we had not made any substantial changes that would have healed my foot. I attribute my miraculous healing, after 12 months of minimal healing, to the changes I made to the foundation of my life by working on my sleep, nutrition, physical activity, stress levels, and relationships.

Not only did my foot heal, but the rest of my body began to heal as well. The stifling fatigue of the past decade, which I had attributed to my CVID, started improving. Since I had more energy and my foot was finally healed, I started doing Pilates again after an eight-year hiatus. I began walking and hiking with friends. Also, I started rollerblading again, which had been a hobby I enjoyed as a teenager and in my twenties. I found that when I was physically active, I wanted to fuel my body with more whole foods. Since I was feeling better, I felt more confident and started socializing more and reconnecting with old friends.

In my new job in the obesity medicine clinic at the VA hospital, I found myself using the pillars of Lifestyle Medicine to counsel my patients not only on weight management but also on how to improve their overall health. This discussion of lifestyle is my favorite part of the visit with my patients. By early summer 2022, I knew I needed to fill in the gaps in my LM education and pursue certification. I found studying for the Lifestyle Medicine board exam enjoyable. I loved learning new pieces of information that I could apply to improve not only the lives of my patients but also myself. I was excited that I passed the board exam in the fall of 2022. I entered 2023 committed to my purpose of embodying the pillars of lifestyle medicine and spreading that knowledge to my patients.

Now, it has been almost two and a half years since the day I broke my foot. I am in a better place in all aspects of my life. In some ways, I feel like I have a variety of fractures to thank for my life makeover. COVID cracked open society as we knew it and forced me into complete solitude. This isolation forced me to truly examine my life and how I wanted to live it and have a meaningful career. My foot fracture was a glimpse into the future of my health if I continued to ignore my nutrition and physical activity. The ruptured water heater and ensuing flood and cleanup demonstrated that starting over did not have to be stressful or daunting but could be liberating.

I threw away not only my ruined belongings but my old, limiting beliefs. My CVID diagnosis did not have to mean that I was an unhealthy person. While my regular immunoglobulin therapy prevents me from infection and getting sick, it is not a guarantee of wellness or good health. I realized that it was my responsibility to make as many changes to my life as possible and to gift myself with the best health I can achieve. I am far from perfect in my personal practice of lifestyle medicine, but every day I wake up trying to do the best I can. I am excited to see how much more I can improve my life over the next year using the pillars of LM. In contrast, sometimes I think back to my young patient with obesity-induced heart failure. I wonder if he would have been in his precarious medical situation at such a young age if he had a healthcare provider trained in Lifestyle Medicine who could have intervened five to 10 years earlier, and perhaps he may have had a far different and better outcome. My passion is the prevention of diseases and the suffering they cause. I can think of no better form of prevention than the practice of Lifestyle Medicine. I have given the rest of my life to this field for myself, my family, my friends, and my patients. I hope sharing my life story inspires you to change yours.

This chapter is dedicated to my parents, Patty and Bob Hagerich, whose endless love and support has encouraged me to become the best version of myself. Also, to my faithful companion, Charlie, who has been by my side through it all.

About Dr. Kelley Hagerich, MD, MPH, FACP, DipABOM, DipABLM

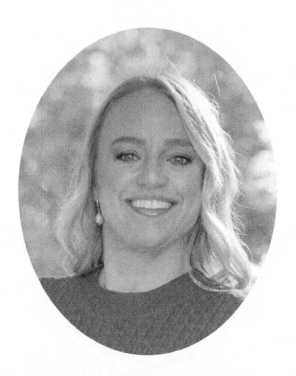

Dr. Kelley Hagerich is quadruple board certified in Internal Medicine, General Preventive Medicine and Public Health, Lifestyle Medicine, and Obesity Medicine. She completed residency programs in Internal Medicine, General Preventive Medicine, and Public Health. While she has always had a strong interest in LM, which she explored during her preventive medicine training, she also recently completed board certification in Lifestyle Medicine to advance her interest in this area. Dr. Hagerich is the national lead physician champion for the Veterans Healthcare System weight management program called the MOVE! program. She also serves as the medical director of the newly developed regional bariatric surgery program based at the VA Palo Alto Healthcare System. Prior to transferring to the VA Palo Alto Healthcare System in January 2022, she spent nine years at the VA San Diego Healthcare System, where she worked as a primary care provider and served as the medical director of the weight management clinic. She was also an Associate Clinical Professor of Medicine at the University of California San Diego (UCSD) School of Medicine, where she taught UCSD medical students and served as a preceptor for the UCSD Internal Medicine residency program.

Instagram: https://www.instagram.com/dr_kelley_hagerich/

Twitter: https://twitter.com/drkhagerich?lang=en

LinkedIn: https://www.linkedin.com/in/kelley-hagerich-md-mph-facp-dabom-13896129

Watch an interview with the co-author:

Co-Author spotlight
DR. KELLEY HAGERICH

Scan Me

8

LIFESTYLE MEDICINE AS SELF-CARE

Teresa Hardisty, MD, FAAP, DipABLM

"Be gentle with yourself. You are a child of the universe, no less than the trees and the stars."

— Max Ehrmann

L et's start with love . . . Who in your past has helped you feel loved? Who and what do you love? Who loves you today? These questions are the core of our human existence and are also woven into the practice of Lifestyle Medicine (LM).

For me, the six pillars of Lifestyle Medicine—healthful nutrition, daily physical activity, restful sleep, stress resiliency, meaningful relationships, and avoiding risky habits/substances—are echoes from the past in my grandmothers' voices and my family's experiences. As the child of European immigrants, I was raised in the home of the free in Virginia Beach by my brilliant but stern Austrian father and my loving but overly trusting English mother without many of the traditional American habits. We visited our relatives overseas regularly, where we ate from the garden, went on long nature walks, and read books together. My childhood memories include endless days at the beach, meals enjoyed around a picnic blanket on a mountaintop, and bedtime stories experienced while folded into my grandmother's embrace. Although my family was not able to protect me from the chaos and challenges of real life, I felt loved and well-connected to my near and far-flung relatives. In the process, I learned early on to take care of myself and, thankfully, was able to follow the paths of my mother and my grandmother to become a physician.

From my childhood experiences, it was a natural fit to choose primary care as a medical specialty. The LM pillars are foundational priorities, especially in pediatrics, with our focus on family relationships and preventive care. Having practiced general pediatrics since 1989 and practiced as well on my own four dear children, I have promoted good health habits and natural remedies in parallel with medicines and procedures when needed. In the course of my own life, this strategy has helped me to maintain relatively good health. It has also helped me weather many significant storms, such as family divorce and separation, brushes with traumatic childhood experiences, and struggling with the challenges of addiction in multiple of my family members.

Some of you readers may know that "self-care" is one of the most empowering aspects of recovery, whether recovery of the addict, recovery from trauma, or recovery by family members affected by addiction and trauma. Not coincidentally, the topics of self-care are exactly the same as the pillars of LM.

For me, self-care starts with self-acceptance. It begins with self-respect and self-awareness and, more importantly, the experience of feeling lovable. Self-care allows me to prioritize my own time, my choices, and my health, even when life seems crazy and when others are not taking care of themselves. Self-acceptance also lays the foundation for me to accept others just as they are, not needing to judge or change even those I love. Self-care ultimately means self-love, and as a LM physician, that is my goal: *To help people learn to love themselves.*

Practically speaking, the implementation of LM is based on health coaching as the main method for promoting behavior change. We, LM practitioners, find what motivates people and frame their choices in the context of their own real life. When people are ready, we use the "5 A's" of motivational interviewing: Assess a health concern, Advise about the science linking the concern to LM, Ask about readiness, Assist with making a small goal, and Arrange follow-up for accountability and support. Health coaching is a well-documented strategy for sparking behavior change. It is also a natural expression of open-mindedness and acceptance, which helps people become curious about their choices. When I counsel individuals about LM, I teach the science of how the LM pillars affect their particular health concerns. I accept them without judgment or my own agenda for them. When they are ready, I offer to help them make an action plan. Sometimes, it is as simple as teaching a breathing exercise to the teen with needle phobia. Incorporating the principles of recovery into this dialogue has made it easier for me to communicate that we do not need to be defined by our past or by other people's expectations. We become aware of a problem, accept the reality of our situation, and then choose our action/response. We become curious about the possibilities.

Besides my natural inclination to follow the pillars of LM (quite imperfectly still, by the way) and the beautiful overlap of Lifestyle Medicine with the self-care and self-acceptance promoted by my recovery experience, this strategy has even helped deepen my faith journey. I have always known that I am part of something bigger than myself, whether it be my connection to my loving family, the awe I feel when surrounded by nature, or my relationship with my church. Over the course of time, I have come to realize that the practice of LM is an opportunity for me to love my neighbors as myself. I meet others with open-mindedness and gratitude and start by loving them exactly as they are. I recognize that when my brother or sister does well, our community does well and that what happens to others affects me profoundly.

When my work partner, Dr. Cherie Chu, first mentioned LM certification to me in 2019, I felt a light bulb go off in my head. I came to really see that these people spoke my language; we are a tribe of people who strive to help ourselves while helping others. In medicine, the temptation is to put our own needs on the back burner, to be a perfectionist, not just to get into medical school but in our entire career. Add the impossibility of taking care of everyone perfectly at every turn, the crushing time commitment of the electronic medical record, and the long hours, and one can easily see why healthcare is in crisis mode, with provider burnout shrinking our ranks on a daily basis. And that was before the COVID-19 pandemic!

Currently, my clinical practice of LM is with individual patients and their family members. I address patient concerns one-on-one, such as pediatric obesity, prediabetes, anxiety, insomnia, and intestinal complaints, among other issues. In addition, I lead the LM program at our large multispecialty group, where I have helped develop customized in-house continuing medical education (CME) for physicians, dieticians, nurses, and other staff members. I represent Sharp Healthcare on the American College of Lifestyle Medicine (ACLM) Health Systems Council, where we share best practices and resources to bring to our local practices. Within our own organization, we also are now doing group visits and building a website for accessing educational and clinical services. We have a strong emphasis on provider and staff support. Additionally, I enjoy speaking and writing about the field of LM.

With the fellow voices of the LM team at Sharp Rees Stealy Medical Group and Sharp Healthcare, we partner with local and national leaders to actually make a difference. One last and perhaps most meaningful way that LM inspires us is when we realize that being kind to ourselves as individuals strengthens our community, which in turn is good for our environment and our planet.

So let's get back to "Who loves YOU?" You might answer that someone now or in your past has loved you, but I hope you might also say that you love yourself. Maybe you can even feel that spark of holy love inside yourself that unites us all. My prayer is that by incorporating the pillars of Lifestyle Medicine and practicing self-care/self-love, you and I can live our best lives. We can be the best versions of ourselves and really be present for the people and the experiences that lie ahead.

———◄○►———

This chapter is dedicated to my grandmother, Lady Iris Gaddum, who was my 1st role model of how healers heal.

———◄○►———

About Dr. Teresa Hardisty, MD, FAAP, DipABLM

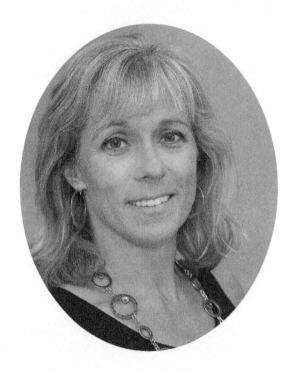

Dr. Teresa Hardisty graduated from the University of California San Diego School of Medicine in 1986 and is board certified in Pediatrics and Lifestyle Medicine. She lives with her husband in San Diego, California. She is the proud mother of four wonderful adult children and grandmother of three amazing grandchildren. In her free time, Dr. Hardisty enjoys traveling, reading, doing yoga, skiing, gardening, watching sunsets, and spending time with friends and family.

Watch an interview with the co-author:

DR. TERESA HARDISTY

Scan Me

9

Considering the Whole Person in the Practice of Medicine

Claudine Holt, MD, MPH, DipABLM, BCC

"Everyone works in the service of man. We doctors work directly on man himself... Our mission is not finished when medicines are no longer of use. We must bring the soul to God."

— St. Gianna Beretta Molla, M.D.

I don't believe in coincidences, and life has confirmed this to me over and over again.

My journey to Lifestyle Medicine (LM) was circuitous, like my journey to becoming a physician. As a child, I actually dreamed of becoming a news anchor/journalist, and my determination led me to pick up the phone to call the local NBC station one day and request to have a chat with my favorite news anchor, who graciously obliged. However, when the Persian Gulf War broke out, I decided I wasn't cut out for journalism if it meant traveling to war zones! It wasn't until high school that the first seeds of becoming a doctor were planted.

I entered university as a pre-med major in biology, but my right-brain creative side won out over my science-loving left brain, and I switched majors to English literature without giving much thought to what I would do with my degree. Upon graduation, I had two very different job opportunities: teaching first grade or working on the public health team of a trade association for chemical companies. This time my left brain won out. It was this job that rekindled my interest in medicine and public health and led me to start volunteering in the intensive care unit (ICU) of a Level 1 trauma center in Washington, DC. After volunteering for a short time, I was hired to work in the ICU while continuing my pre-med studies.

The year I applied to medical school, I sustained a 3rd-degree ankle sprain and fibula fracture, which sidelined me for several weeks as I recovered from ankle fixation surgery and then a hardware removal surgery the following year. During that time, my weight steadily increased as the bad eating habits I developed in college finally caught up with me (and I wasn't able to be active to balance it out). But in hindsight, I can see that I was emotionally traumatized by the injury. I likely went into shock when I looked down and saw my left foot dangling from my ankle because I didn't feel any pain until hours later. I remember feeling guilty for needing my family to take care of me and help me get to appointments because they were already working hard and stretched thin.

By the time I moved to Columbus, OH, for medical school a few months later, my weight was higher than ever, and I felt self-conscious. For the first two years of medical school, I went back and forth between different providers at the Student Health Clinic as well as the nurse practitioner back home in Maryland to figure out why my weight continued to increase. It was clearly more than just being sedentary after the ankle fracture since I was back on my feet by this point. But time and time again, I was simply told, "Eat less, exercise more."

Finally, after returning from Geneva, Switzerland, where I interned at the World Health Organization (WHO) for eight weeks, my body sent me a clear signal that I couldn't ignore. I was back in Ohio and starting my third-year clinical rotations when, amid all this excitement and stress, I had an irregular cycle for the first time in my life. I immediately knew something was terribly wrong. I scheduled an appointment with the gynecologist at Student Health Clinic, and she suspected something hormonal was going on. She gave me a progesterone challenge test which resolved the issue. The following month, I had an irregular cycle again, and she obtained blood work that confirmed a hormonal disorder.

Although there was a brief mention of diet and exercise, I was immediately started on medications to try to balance my hormones and prevent the development of other serious conditions like diabetes. But the medications made me nauseous, and I became concerned about the long-term side effects. I spent several years trying different diets and medications to help manage my symptoms and prevent the development of metabolic syndrome, but nothing seemed to work long-term.

While working my first job as an attending physician, I discovered life coaching in 2013, and it turned my world upside down in the best way. For the first time, I understood how I was actually "at cause" in my life instead of "at effect." I learned about the cognitive triad and how my thoughts influenced my feelings, and how my feelings fueled the actions I was taking (or not taking). I started to experience a real transformation in my mindset and thinking, which eventually led to weight loss. However, those changes didn't fully stick until I learned more about the mind-body connection through somatic (body-based) coaching. I learned that healing isn't just something that happens from the neck up but involves the whole person—mind, body, and spirit.

I wondered why no one ever taught me this information and why this isn't something we learn in school. Certainly, as physicians, we should understand the mind-body connection better than anyone, right? I wanted to shout my newfound knowledge from the rooftops and help other people, so I decided to become a life coach. It was around the time of being coached and becoming a coach that I learned about Lifestyle

Medicine (LM) from a couple of work colleagues who were pursuing board certification. Once I learned about the six pillars, the light bulbs went off, and it was a full-circle moment for me. I could see that everything I had experienced until this point in my personal life, physical health, emotional well-being, spirituality, and career could be framed and understood through the lens of the six pillars of LM—which meant I could use this knowledge to empower my patients.

By the end of 2022, I had lost over 40 pounds through intermittent fasting, limiting flour and sugar, and focusing on whole foods. I also purchased a spin bike which I use 4-6 days per week, and I do barre for stretching and strengthening. My Catholic faith and daily spiritual practice are an important part of my life, and I also have a 1:1 coach. My goal is to lead by example by embodying what I teach my patients and coaching clients.

In 2022, I also completed the LM course, attended my first LM conference, and became board certified in LM. One of my colleagues, who is also board certified in Lifestyle Medicine, and I are piloting a LM program in our department, and my clinical impression is that we are already seeing amazing results in the first few months, such as weight loss, decrease in reflux scores, and reduced use of anti-reflux medications.

Medicine is as much an art as a science, and Lifestyle Medicine has given me the opportunity to combine coaching and medical skills in a new and exciting way. The old medical paradigm teaches clinicians to look at patients as discrete organ systems that become diseased. We don't usually consider mental and emotional factors until other etiologies have been ruled out. The reality is that patients want us to see them *and* treat them as a whole person. They want less siloed care and are more in favor of an integrative approach. They want us to meet them where they are and create treatment plans *with* them that are challenging but achievable. Most importantly, they want us to believe in them—and their capacity to heal—even when they don't fully believe in themselves.

(Disclaimer: The thoughts and opinions expressed in this chapter are the author's and do not necessarily represent the views of her employer or academic institution.)

This chapter is dedicated to my mother, Shirley, whose unceasing prayers provided the light that guided my path.

About Dr. Claudine Holt, MD, MPH, DipABLM, BCC

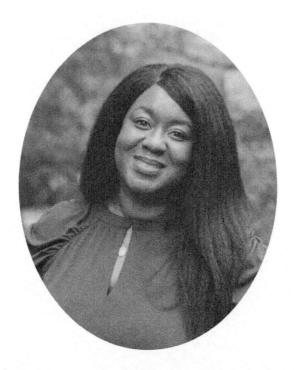

Dr. Claudine Holt is board certified in Occupational and Environmental Medicine and Lifestyle Medicine. She received her undergraduate degree from Georgetown University and completed her MPH and residency at Johns Hopkins University. She is an assistant professor at the Selikoff Centers for Occupational Medicine at the Mount Sinai School of Medicine in New York.

She believes in a holistic and integrative approach to healing that addresses the mind, body, and spirit. Beyond her medical training, she is a board-certified coach (BCC), feminine embodiment coach, professional certified coach through the Life Coach School, and has additional certifications in integrative somatic trauma and clinical hypnotherapy.

In her private coaching practice, The Embodied MD, she teaches women how to stop gaslighting themselves so they can recover from burnout without feeling guilty.

Website: https://www.theembodiedmd.com

LinkedIn: https://www.linkedin.com/in/claudine-holt-m-d-0755425/

Instagram: https://www.instagram.com/theembodiedmd/

Watch an interview with the co-author:

DR. CLAUDINE HOLT

Scan Me

10

THE WIS(ER) VEGETARIAN

Julia M. Huber, MD, DipABLM, TIPC

"We are all just walking each other home."

— Ram Dass

"You are such a DUMB vegetarian!" These were harsh words for me, a tree-hugging clerk cashing out granola in a health food store in the early 1990s. I was ringing out one of the mountain climbing jocks who worked at the hiking supply store a few doors down. Like me, he was also in his mid-20s, a gangly guy who came in each morning for his cup of Joe. I could feel my little round face grow hot and flushed, and I was irritated. Plus, I was feeling really fat that day, and he wasn't helping. Not a great start to a Monday morning. He saw what I ate for breakfast: bread with lurid wads of "all-natural" margarine. Sometimes I would sit in the back, pull out a jar of the stuff, and cram it in on my breaks. Hey, the animals are okay, and I'm a healthy vegetarian! He had caught me red-handed and was merciless but spot on. I truly had no clue what I was shoving into my body and couldn't figure out why I weighed more than what was healthy for me because, gosh, I wasn't eating meat or desserts. At minimum wage, I couldn't afford new jeans, so each day, I had to gasp to zip and button them up before donning my little blue work apron. I wished my eating and weight conundrum weren't so obvious to him and wished he had just kept his thoughts to himself, but fat shaming seems to be part of our modern culture—so this was just another day at work.

This episode took place the year before I applied and was accepted to medical school. Between shifts at the natural foods venue, I could be found at the local rescue squad driving ambulances and caring for patients in my hometown as an EMT-ST (emergency medical technician - shock trauma). If you were one of the regulars there, you got a nickname: there was "Spark" for the very slow-moving and deliberate colleague who pretty much shuffled to any emergency; "Bugman," who worked for the local exterminator company when he wasn't saving human lives; and my nickname was "Granola Head." It was a given that I would show up at the squad house for my shift with slightly stale "health food" donated from the store as an alternative to the sausage and gravy biscuits with eggs cooked up for the crew most mornings. So it kind of stung to be called "dumb" about my diet, especially since I had a reputation among my peers for being so healthy. But, once I got over his negativity, I could see that my customer's point was well taken. I looked around me at the shelves closest to the checkout counter: everything we sold at the store was "all-natural," meaning no preservatives or artificial colors, but our fastest-moving treats all were essentially full of empty calories, such as crispy potato chips and juice-flavored sodas laden with fructose syrup, "energy" bars with calories and not much nutritional value.

I went home that night and thought about what he said. No, I didn't have a background in nutrition. Other than knowing that I was eating lower on the food chain as a vegetarian and being a track runner in high school and college (so a little bit into the fitness world), and having a meditation practice, I hadn't deeply considered the wider realm of wellness as it relates to healthful food choices as well as the far-reaching implications for the community and the globe.

Why be vegetarian? Is it really that healthy, after all? Why does it matter? In high school, I read an eye-opening novel called _The Jungle_ by Upton Sinclair, which depicted slaughterhouse conditions in Chicago around the 1900s. I also grew up in rural Virginia, where my family raised and sold lambs for slaughter, and as such knew firsthand that for philosophical and moral reasons, I didn't want to eat meat. But what about the nutritional aspect? And what about my goal in my late 20s to begin my trajectory as a physician—as someone who learns about and educates their patients about health? I had a ton of questions.

During my ambulance runs, I started seeing predictable patterns: the patients with end-stage cardiac disease, more often than not, also had hypertension, high cholesterol, diabetes, a high body mass index (BMI), and often had to be extricated with rescue equipment just to get them out of their residence. I quietly certified in rope and mountain rescue so we, along with our crew and the fire department, could figure out how to extricate large patients from their residence swiftly and safely. Many of our patients lived in homes that exuded the odor of old fried grease, sometimes clinging in gritty droplets even in their living rooms. Some patients were so oversized compared to their residence that on one occasion, the Fire Department had to cut out the wall of a patient's narrow trailer just to get them loaded up and out to the ER. My heart broke for these patients and their families.

The lack of access to healthy food and healthy housing, coupled with the overall lack of education about these issues, was clearly causing misery and truncating lives. We didn't judge, we just tried to help the best we could. It was a head-on dive into the world of poverty and, at least in my hometown, one which seemed inextricably linked to cultural issues, racial issues, and community access issues. One of our important tasks as medics was to grab a plastic bag and throw all the patient medications into it for the ER staff to review on patient arrival; it was usually a large plastic grocery bag we filled with dozens of pills and patches and inhalers. Fast forward, and I was to witness this over and over as an emergency physician for several decades, noticing the pale yellow rings around a patient's iris as we spoke, then the unsurprising blood draw with the clear grease or "lipids" rising to the top of the test tube, further evidence of their hyperlipidemia, followed by the grossly high confirmatory lab results.

Between my cashier shifts in 1990, I began to expand my reading, digging deeper into what we eat and the far-reaching implications not only for each individual and their communities but for the world. I began to devour the book offerings from the health food store while on my breaks at the granola shop. There was Fit for Life, liquid diets, the cabbage soup diet, cottage cheese diet, and numerous others. It was hard to make sense of trendy reads. I did find some encouraging books, such as Francis Moore Lappé's _Diet for a Small Planet_ and Molly Katzen's now classic _The Moosewood Cookbook_, which ushered in the era of yummy-tasting vegetarian fare. I watched firsthand as customers bought fad diet books and grocery items to match them, but there was also a trend toward lower-fat diets based on the work of early visionaries such as Dr. Dean Ornish. Now, I at least knew to ditch some of the fat I was eating, and the weight came off, although the memory of stinging criticism remained.

There was something earthshaking about _Diet for a Small Planet_ by Francis Moore Lappé. Her messaging was really clear and, like _The Jungle_ did when it was first published, Moore Lappé broke open the conversation about the business of raising and slaughtering animals for protein consumption and its far-reaching impact on the world's resources. She coupled that with education about plant proteins, how to match up beans and grains for a more complete diet, tossed in a few recipes crowd-sourced from her friends, and this became the "plant-based Bible" of the late 20th century. As noted in a New York Times article looking back at the legacy left by "The Godmother" of 'Plant-Based' Living, "[v]ege-tarianism in those days was a strange if not heretical way of nourishing oneself . . . Ms. Lappé was 'plant-based' long before the term existed."

I don't recall hearing the term "plant-based" when I entered medical school in the early '90s, and there was no specific nutrition class, but in retrospect, they taught us down to the molecular and cellular level what is behind what we eat in a given day, and how those choices can fre-quently contribute to activating disease states. Thiamine deficiency and alcoholism, as well as B12 deficiency and vegetarianism, were presented in the same lecture. I felt a bit defensive, perhaps triggered by the "dumb vegetarian" accusation from the previous year, which implied that a vegetarian may do ignorant things that hurt their body due to nutritional deficiencies. Sadly, we didn't learn the benefits of vegetarianism at that point.

The Adventist Health Study research was hot off the press, demonstrating that "levels of cholesterol, diabetes, high blood pressure and metabolic syndrome all had the same trend—the closer you are to being a vegetarian, the lower the health risk in these areas." Despite my defensiveness about my lifestyle choices, I focused on doing extra reading about how the individual components of food and how the molecular structure alone can completely alter the course of one's health when one makes healthy and preventive moves early on. I learned more about the literal bonds that form fats, understanding that the location of double bonds between atoms in a type of fat molecule could make it less healthy for humans to consume. Our biochemistry professor, a quirky man with a neat bowtie and a classical way of teaching, linked articles from the New England Journal of Medicine about trans or "bad" fats and advised us not to eat margarine (Mensink et al.). This wasn't "woo-woo" material anymore if it was making it into the lecture hall of a medical school steeped in research and tradition. It amazed me that for all of the fad diets that were so popular, the lay public (including yours truly just a few months prior!) really didn't seem to know about these scientific studies quite yet, even though the first studies came out as early as 1981! (Thomas et al.). Why was this information not in the headlines? It would be another 10 or 15 years before the FDA required trans fats to appear on food labels so Americans could make informed choices (The Nutrition Source).

There were a few glimmers of Lifestyle Medicine (LM) and wellness didactics when we started learning how to analyze laboratory results during first-year medical school pathology lectures. Our professors told us to show up one morning without eating breakfast. They drew fasting blood samples, gave us detailed questionnaires, and a few weeks later, we had our personal and group results to learn to analyze. We looked at our medical school class as a cohort, and without naming names, we could see how many smokers there were (very few!). Several of my peers realized they were perhaps a bit above their BMI for optimal health. We each had a glucometer to take home along with saline in lieu of insulin, and for several weeks we simulated the lifestyle of an insulin-dependent diabetic. We checked our blood sugars multiple times a day using sharp lancets to place a drop of blood on the glucometer and used actual needles and syringes to draw up the saline and self-inject. We had to follow an 1,800-calorie American Diabetes Association (ADA) diet as we were diabetics. The impact was phenomenal. With results in front of them, I saw colleagues lose weight, and several of the smokers stopped smoking. The one peer, who chewed tobacco and dribbled its dark juice into an empty Mountain Dew bottle during lecture, stopped his habit cold turkey, much to everyone's relief. Thinking back, these were the building blocks of the current practice of Lifestyle Medicine, only I didn't quite realize it at the time. I remain grateful that my medical school professors gave me the rigorous scientific training and ability to critically think, analyze, and treat both chronic and acute conditions. I also left with an appreciation for what we ask of one another as colleagues and what we ask of our patients in terms of making choices to live a healthy lifestyle.

As an attending physician, my learning continued. It wasn't until I was an Emergency Physician that I started reading more about circadian rhythms because ours were constantly being jerked around as we went from days to night and back to days again—sometimes several times in a week. The Nurses Health Study findings were beginning to be published. They linked rotating night shifts and other lifestyle choices around food, physical activity, and smoking with diminished longevity and an increase in chronic disease. (For a good summary of these studies, check out https://ajph.aphapublications.org/doi/full/10.2105/AJPH. 2016.303345.). I often thought about my days working in the natural foods store and decided to supplement my reading on nutrition and well-being, despite being in a specialty that focused on acute care. I continued to witness the sad endpoints of chronic disease that I had noticed as an EMT. I don't know how many times I have thought that someone I pronounced dead didn't deserve to die this way. In so many cases, much of their chronic disease could have been prevented or potentially reversed. After about 30 years, this daily onslaught of disease was absolutely heartbreaking.

Meanwhile, I noticed that often patients were fat-shamed and would delay being seen for care until a scenario became a true emergency. The words from the mountaineering jock/customer years ago never ever went away; I knew better than to fat-shamed people and to make them feel "dumb" or less than. We all have our reasons for how we eat, and that's no reason to criticize and denigrate people for being uneducated about their condition. As I continued in my career, I saw our culture and conversations change about vegetarianism and lifestyle choices, but there always seemed to be something missing. With my interest in wellness, it was a natural course for me to become an advocate for physician wellness with my professional association. I became certified as a trauma-informed professional coach so I could work one-on-one with my colleagues privately, often at no charge, as the levels of burnout increased. Many of my physician clients had developed chronic diseases as a response to chronic massive stress, leading them to quit practicing medicine altogether. Several died early, some by suicide, and other issues related to the deep trauma of practicing in what was often labeled a "toxic workplace" scenario. Again, the same thought process repeated in my head: What else could be done to prevent or mitigate these issues so that people can live healthy, joy-filled lives?

Then, COVID happened, lockdown came, and global levels of fear, anxiety, and isolation were at unprecedented highs. I think many of us spent time worrying and wondering how we would survive as a species. I worried the most about my family, community, and colleagues, who were suffering from burnout even more than before. Physician burnout and attrition soon became tantamount to a public health emergency. The isolation of lockdown caused severe damage on emotional levels. We witnessed firsthand how isolation has a negative effect on one's health and well-being, as evidenced by the global uptick in depression and anxiety and frank full-blown PTSD among patients and healthcare professionals alike.

I began to pull together the pieces: the global impact of our community and dietary practices, the science behind a plant-based diet, the impact of shift work on our health, the devastating disconnect of the pandemic, and the cumulative trauma and damage to our bodies, hearts, minds, and souls. It was all riveting. By that point, I was already certified as a trauma-informed yoga instructor, ICF-certified trauma-informed professional coach, and a meditation teacher, but the concept of global wellness still seemed fragmented somehow, even as my coaching clients were starting to ask me about lifestyle choices as a way to prevent or even heal from the effects of COVID.

Enter Lifestyle Medicine! After locating the <u>American College of Lifestyle Medicine (ACLM)</u> online, I started reading about the Six Pillars of LM, and it simply made sense. Using evidence-based research, American Board of Lifestyle Medicine (ABLM)-certified practitioners knew how to assess a patient for readiness to change, evaluate for risky substances in a nonjudgmental way, and address patients' weight concerns in an open-minded way. By referring to evidence-based guidelines around following a plant-based diet, we were able to avoid being trendy and offer support to patients as part of a community working toward wellness. Add to that essential stress management, guidance around getting in motion, and education around sleep hygiene, as well as advocacy for our deeply human need for social connection for us to live healthy and happy lives, and the world of wellness and the world of "regular" medical practice came together beautifully.

During the COVID-19 lockdown, I turned my gaze to completing the requisite coursework and conferences with the ACLM and passed my board certification with the ABLM. As a health educator and wellness consultant with certification in LM with the ABLM, I feel I can now complement the work of a patient's primary care physician by adding in the six pillars of LM for a more complete, 360 approach toward health to reverse many of the chronic diseases I saw my ER patients dying of, and even getting them off many of their medications!

As for this "dumb" vegetarian? I have so much more to learn. There's always something else we can do to better serve our patients, family, community, and ourselves in wellness. I have agency and boundaries now around negative commentary, whether in the workplace or the private realm. It gives me profound joy to help others shift their perspective and take a stand for living their lives in peace and abundant health. I recognize that medical training has also evolved, and am grateful for the evidence-based critical thinking my medical school instilled in me. Lay people now have easier access to groundbreaking scientific research more than ever before, but I know from my personal and professional experience that it's really helpful to have the added partnership and advocacy of a LM specialist. I have learned that we also need one another to grow in wellness together throughout our lives. My daughters are now almost the same age I was when I was an ambulance driving "Granola Head." We cook plant-based meals together, and as a reminder that I have more to learn, I still have the same blue apron from the natural foods store in my hometown! I continue to learn daily from my interactions with coaching clients, my patients, and from my LM colleagues. I am grateful for the small study group of other physicians from all over the country who prepared together on Zoom for our ABLM certification. They have been colleagues and friends who have supported me professionally and personally as I have faced my share of health issues from COVID. We continue to work together to share knowledge and understanding of LM as the field continues to flourish and grow.

If I learned anything from lockdown and from the studies of LM, it's that health education matters, access to evidence-based information matters, and connection from one human heart to another human heart deeply matters. Do we have a corner on the market? I doubt it. But we do have a beautiful rendering of the puzzle pieces that are a melding of the conversations of those before us, the visionaries like Frances Moore Lappé who have brought the messaging to the public, as well as the many scientists researching the lifestyle choices that prevent chronic disease. I would like to express deep gratitude to Dr. John Kelly for founding the American College of Lifestyle Medicine. I would like to think I am not so "dumb" anymore. I am certainly much more at ease in my body and have a deeper comprehension of what impacts my well-being as a patient with a chronic disease as well as a physician and human being.

I recently spent two weeks on a retreat in Morocco with Dr. Omid Safi, a Professor of Islamic Studies at Duke University and a Sufi scholar. He said that when Sufis ask, "How are you?" they use the word "*qalb*" in lieu of the word "you," which references a person's inner heart space, or their essence. In other words, they are asking, "How is your heart?" My hope for all of us in this beautiful but sometimes disjointed world is that we look at one another without judgment and truly ask one another, "How ARE you, really?" And be available to listen to the true answer as we connect on that level as human beings. As our Surgeon General, Dr. Vivek Murthy writes in his book *Together: The Healing Power of a Human Connection in a Sometimes Lonely World* (p. 279):

> "Dear Ones, May you inhabit a world that puts people at the center, where everyone feels they belong. Where compassion is universal, and kindness is exchanged with whole-hearted generosity for all. The most important thing we wish for you is a life filled with love—love that is given and received with a full heart. Love is at the heart of living a connected life. Choose love, we tell you. Always."

Thank you for this opportunity to write about Wellness and Lifestyle Medicine.

———◆◇◆———

Dedicated to my beautiful daughters,
Maya and Asha.

———◆◇◆———

References:

Sinclair, U. (2010). *The Jungle*. OUP Oxford.

Lappé, F. M. (2021). *Diet for a Small Planet (Revised and Updated)*. National Geographic Books.

Katzen, M. (2014). *The Moosewood Cookbook: 40th Anniversary Edition*. Ten Speed Press.

Kurutz, S. (2021, November 20). The Godmother of 'Plant-Based' Living. *The New York Times*. https://www.nytimes.com/2021/11/20/styl e/frances-moore-lappe-diet-small-planet.html.

Adventist Health Study | Adventist Health Study. https://adventisthea lthstudy.org/.

Findings for Lifestyle, Diet & Disease | Adventist Health Study. https:// adventisthealthstudy.org/studies/AHS-2/findings-lifestyle-diet-disease.

Mensink, R. P., & Katan, M. B. (1990). Effect of Dietary Trans Fatty Acids on High-Density and Low-Density Lipoprotein Cholesterol Levels in Healthy Subjects. *The New England Journal of Medicine*, *323*(7), 439–445. https://doi.org/10.1056/nejm199008163230703.

Thomas, L. H., Jones, P. B., Winter, J., & Smith, H. (1981). Hydrogenated oils and fats: the presence of chemically-modified fatty acids in human adipose tissue. *The American Journal of Clinical Nutrition, 34*(5), 877–886. https://doi.org/10.1093/ajcn/34.5.877.

Shining the Spotlight on Trans Fats. (2021, March 8). The Nutrition Source. https://www.hsph.harvard.edu/nutritionsource/what-should -you-eat/fats-and-cholesterol/types-of-fat/transfats/.

American Diabetes Association | Research, Education, Advocacy. (n.d.). https://diabetes.org/.

Nurses' Health Study |. https://nurseshealthstudy.org/.

Morabia, A. (2016). 120 000 Nurses Who Shook Public Health. *American Journal of Public Health, 106*(9), 1528–1529. https://doi.org/10. 2105/ajph.2016.303345.

Home - American College of Lifestyle Medicine. (2023, May 9). American College of Lifestyle Medicine. https://lifestylemedicine.org/.

General, O. O. T. S. (2022, March 24). *Vice Admiral Vivek H. Murthy, MD, MBA.* HHS.gov. https://www.hhs.gov/about/leadership/vivek -murthy.html.

Murthy, V. H., MD. (2020). *Together: The Healing Power of Human Connection in a Sometimes Lonely World.* HarperCollins.

About Dr. Julia Huber, MD, DipABLM, TIPC

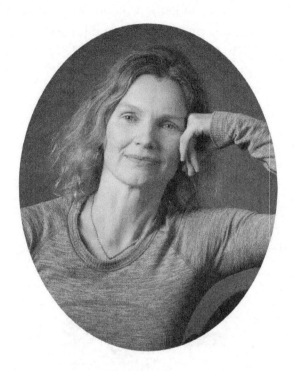

Dr. Julia M. Huber is a wellness consultant and trauma-informed professional coach who works with physicians and other professionals who are suffering from burnout and who are ready to make a significant change in their lives, particularly in the years leading up to retirement. https://juliamariehuberMD.com.

She is boarded in Emergency Medicine as well as Lifestyle Medicine and has an online telemedicine practice via Heal Is Health, https://healish ealth.com.

As an ICF-certified coach with over 15 years of coaching experience, she also has advanced certification as a trauma-informed professional coach via Lodestar (https://www.lodestarpc.com). She is a graduate of Bryn Mawr College, with a major in Spanish Literature, and is a graduate of the University of Virginia School of Medicine. She lives in Lexington, Kentucky, with her family, where she completed a residency in

Emergency Medicine, and she grew up a little south of Charlottesville, Virginia. In her spare time, she gardens, cooks, meditates, and often hikes locally and treks overseas. Her most memorable trip thus far has been the Camino de Santiago in Spain, which she walked once solo in 2019, then again with her two daughters in 2021.

Watch an interview with the co-author:

Co-Author spotlight
DR. JULIA HUBER

Scan Me

*"People think about a diet . . . And so our diet is really . . .
we're feeding one another. We're feeding one another **hope**.
We're feeding one another **vision**. We're feeding one another
wellness. And that's part of our diet if you wish."*

— Dr. Julia Huber

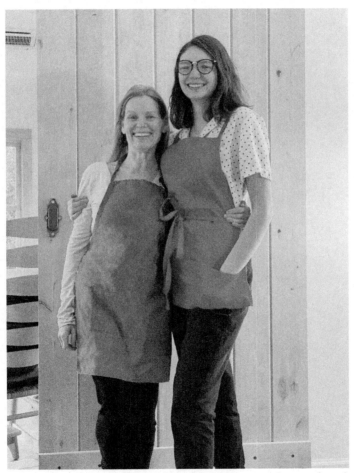

*Dr. Julia Huber with her daughter, Maya, taking a break
from cooking together in 2020!*

11

A SECOND CHANCE – THE WHOLE HEALTH JOURNEY

Geetha Kamath MD, FACP, DipABLM, DipABOM

"A journey of a thousand miles begins with a single step."
— Lao Tsu

In April of 1998, I was a successful rising obstetrician from India who moved to the USA after marrying the love of my life. Being a young, enthusiastic, vibrant happy-go-lucky person, I lived a life full of hustle-bustle in a crowded city in India, and then, overnight, I moved to a small farming town with a population of 3,000 or less in the Midwest, which became my new home. My husband was finishing his job contract there for a couple more years. The relocation came with surprises, both pleasant and shocking, but being an extrovert, I made friends with the locals and senior citizens. I made the best of the cultural exchange and developed new joys and experiences in the small town. To be honest, being away from family and adapting to a new culture was pretty challenging, in spite of all the newfound happiness. I found myself with extra time on my hands in the new small town compared to being the busy gynecologist and teaching doctor I had been until then. There were other unique stressors, the perceived stress of having to start a family with a biological clock ticking and having to study intensely to apply for retraining and licensing to be able to practice as a physician in the United States. It was anything but a piece of cake. These changes are the backdrop of my journey into wellness and lifestyle medicine two decades later.

My lifestyle had changed overnight from being a busy physician and active all day to being a person who sat at home studying for endless hours for the next several months, with breaks for socializing with the new friends I had made best of volunteering at the local public school. My new friends and culture entertained me with wonderful home-baked loaves of bread with butter and delicacies of pastries and pies, and I had access to gallons of ice cream, sodas, and chips. These had all been special treats and bite-size while I had lived in India, perhaps eaten only on special occasions. Now, I had full access to these treats to easily reach out to as a way to deal with the stress of studying. While I was soon blessed with a beautiful baby girl, the pregnancy, lifestyle changes, sitting and studying, stress, along with hormonal changes contributed to a good bit of weight gain during pregnancy and gestational diabetes. Despite being a physician, I considered these pregnancy-related issues that would go away and continued with my mindless eating and lack of a healthy lifestyle.

Throughout medical school, I had learned about diseases and how to treat them, with little education on how lifestyle contributes to chronic diseases and how they could be easily mitigated through healthy choices. My unhealthy lifestyle continued for several years while I focused on and completed my internal medicine training, which was an even more stressful period for me. There was no time for self-care practices, especially 20 years ago when there were no limits to how long the trainees worked. There were days I would be in the hospital for 24–30 hours straight.

While being the resilient person I was, with the support of my colleagues, family, and friends, I overcame many stressful situations during that period. I graduated successfully, joined as a full-time practicing physician at a university medical school, and had two more children in the interim. My husband and I had moved away for training to the East Coast and subsequently decided to move back to the Midwest.

When I changed jobs and joined the VA system, I saw my patients' struggles with chronic diseases like diabetes, hypertension, arthritis, obesity, depression, and PTSD that were managed with multiple medications and procedures. Unfortunately, the focus was not to cure but manage; they would improve for short periods, then flare up and, many a time, worsen or have side effects from their medications or procedures. I started feeling helpless and felt I had to do more than just prescribe pills and offer referrals for procedures to put a Band-Aid on their issue. I felt I had little expertise to advise about nutrition beyond the generic "eat healthy, eat less, exercise more" advice. Patients with back and knee issues usually told me how difficult it was to exercise. How could I get them to achieve 150 minutes of weekly exercise needed to be healthy? I knew I needed to be better educated on these issues to help my patients and guide them and also for my own health.

This was my turning point when I explored my resources and the Whole Health program initiative by the VA health system. The Whole Health program was more aligned with starting the journey of long-term healing and finding a way of life that was more meaningful. I studied and was certified in Obesity Medicine, which focuses on obesity medications, surgery, and lifestyle changes to help with obesity-related health issues. During this time, a dear friend introduced me to Lifestyle Medicine (LM) and all the resources and training provided through the American College of Lifestyle Medicine (ACLM). I joined forces with her and a few like-minded physician friends who were also interested in advocating and promoting healthy behavior in their practice. We studied together during the COVID-19 pandemic via Zoom and passed the certification for Lifestyle Medicine. As part of training, we had to do a practicum aligned with lifestyle medicine pillars. We had the choice to be the subject ourselves for this case study. This requirement to pass allowed me to practice what I planned to preach and have firsthand knowledge of the challenges and ease of incorporating lifestyle changes. Did I mention I very much needed to improve my own health trajectory (that was otherwise leading me down the path of being a diabetic with plantar fasciitis, back pain, sleep issues, and weight issues) with the backdrop of the stress of being a full-time physician, and mother of three young kids—to say the least?

The journey of a lifetime began with that single step of eating more nutrient-dense whole food plant-based meals, cutting out processed foods and sugary beverages, avoiding mindless snacking on chips, learning to walk away from the cookies and cakes at work, and the processed lunch foods at the cafeteria.

I started making it a point to have one to two servings of a variety of vegetables, steamed, stew, or salad that I fixed the night before for lunch and dinner, and eat two fruits every day. I started carrying a water bottle and tracked my daily water intake. Better sleep routines meant setting an alarm to turn off my laptop and other devices an hour before bed and an attempt to add daily bite-sized self-care and mindfulness practices for stress management like 2-3 minutes of stretching or deep breaths, were made a priority in spite of my busy day. I requested and got a standing desk at work. I started taking the time to keep in touch and visit friends and family regularly, either in person or via phone calls. These changes, along with medications as needed, significantly helped improve my overall health and well-being.

Thus the six pillars of lifestyle medicine (nutrition, sleep, social connections, physical activity, stress management, and avoiding addictive foods/substances) now became my strength and support on my lifelong path to heal my body and spirit.

I realized what I had been missing and how it felt so good to feel alive, well, and thrive rather than just surviving day to day. Given this beautiful self-care experiment, I became a big believer in spreading knowledge and resources to all my patients, family, and friends. I stepped into my new role as a teaching physician to the next generation of medical students, resident trainees, and fellowship trainees in how to implement these concepts into patient care. I am the wellness champion for the state chapter and give many well-received lectures and workshops for students and staff at my institution and state and national conferences on self-care and wellness. This is the gift that keeps on giving – like the wonderful saying: "Feed a man [or person] a fish, you feed him for a day; teach a man to fish, you feed him for a lifetime." My kids are teenagers and in their 20s, and they have seen me lead by example at home and practice a healthy lifestyle. Two out of three of them have chosen to be vegetarian for ethical and health benefits.

The Lifestyle Medicine curriculum is gaining momentum due to many reasons, including the rising cost of healthcare, patients' poor quality of life (despite advances in medicine with medications and procedures), the rising global changes of chronic diseases that have helped prolong life but not necessarily promote quality of life. A significant turning point was noted in the last few years when COVID-19 infections caused several deaths globally and noticeably more in people who were considered high risk due to chronic illnesses like diabetes, obesity, and heart disease. The common thread to fix and prevent these illnesses lies in long-term healthy practices of nutrition, sleep, stress management, and disease prevention in the first place. It is now well proven that your genetics/genes are not your destiny, but your dinner (diet) is. Champions of lifestyle, like renowned cardiologist Dr. Dean Ornish, well-known researcher Dr. Colin Campbell, nutrition advocate Dr. Michael Gregor, and several others, have scientifically studied the benefits of lifestyle practices for decades. They have helped save and improve numerous patients' lives and made it their mission to bring this to the limelight through various nonprofit and altruistic activities.

I am fortunate to share my journey with you all and be a part of this milestone shift in the approach to chronic disease and healthcare with a focus on prevention rather than trying to shut the door after the horse is out of the barn when it comes to chronic illness.

I have had the joy of telling several patients they no longer need their blood pressure medication and that their diabetes is now in remission, reducing or stopping insulin injections for several people with diabetes who no longer require it to maintain their blood sugars. I cherish hearing the joy of one patient telling me he can now ride a bike and play basketball with his son. The young man, who had severe anxiety from being 100 lbs heavier prior, and now being able to walk into the grocery store and enjoy shopping on his own. Another patient shared she no longer needed her hip replaced immediately after losing weight and is now able to walk into my office without her walker for the first time in several years. Yet another patient, a young lady who had struggled with infertility, came in a year later with her baby in the stroller. These stories will probably be the chapters for my next book.

Let me finish by saying habits are hard to change and need a lot of support, persistence, and resources that lifestyle medicine provides, including the practical skills and tools needed to make the change. Our life and lifestyle changes are like a marathon, not a sprint. We must approach this with a mindset of making progress rather than aiming for perfection. Lifestyle changes need resources and support at a personal, community, and public health level with measures to smooth the path for change. With the recent White House convention and the pledge by the American College of Lifestyle Medicine and several other organizations to commit to this cause, I am confident and excited to be part of this change in healthcare.

This chapter is my humble offering and token of gratitude to the vast universe, which has provided me with lessons, purpose, and essence of living in various forms, challenges, and opportunities, and helped evolve into a lifetime of growth and transformation!

Additional Learning Resources:

Greger, M. *Nutrition Facts*. Nutrition Facts. https://nutritionfacts.org.

Ackerman, C. E., MA. (2023). What Is Positive Psychology & Why Is It Important? *PositivePsychology.com*. https://positivepsychology.com/what-is-positive-psychology-definition/.

Mozaffarian, D. (2016). Dietary and Policy Priorities for Cardiovascular Disease, Diabetes, and Obesity. *Circulation*, *133*(2), 187–225. https://doi.org/10.1161/circulationaha.115.018585.

About Dr. Geetha Kamath MD, FACP, DipABLM, DipABOM

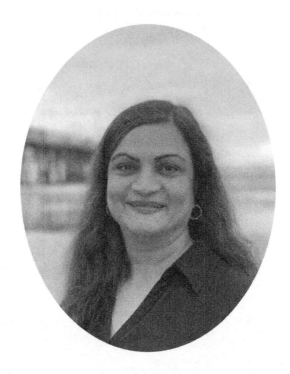

Dr. Geetha Kamath is triple board certified in Internal Medicine, Obesity Medicine, and Lifestyle Medicine and currently is faculty for medical students, residents, and endocrinology and nutrition fellowship training programs at the University of Missouri Kansas City, Kansas City, Missouri.

Having lived in India and completed her medical school and an Obstetrics and Gynecology residency in India, she has seen the challenges of malnutrition and high infant mortality rates.

She is also familiar with the benefits of herbs and plant-based whole foods, the role of nutrition (Ayurveda), and yoga in health and well-being. Her additional certification in Lifestyle and Obesity Medicine has helped her care for patients in a holistic manner and has been rewarding in many ways. As part of self-care and work-life balance, she loves spending time with her family, traveling, gardening, and catching up with old friends as well as meeting new people on her travels. She loves tasting and trying new whole food plant-based recipes from different cultures across the globe.

LinkedIn: https://www.linkedin.com/in/geetha-s-kamath

Watch an interview with the co-author:

Co-Author spotlight
DR. GEETHA KAMATH

 Scan Me

12

"So, Where Do You Get Your Protein?"

Mitika Kanabar MD, MPH, FASAM, DipABLM

"It's more preferable to do your own responsibility imperfect-ly than others' perfectly."

— The Bhagavad Gita

Going through our lives, we all have different experiences in childhood, teenage, young adulthood, and then real "adulting," so to speak. One of the foremost adulting tasks is meal prepping, 'What will we eat today or this week?' We come up with some options—ranging from gourmet-looking meals to takeout, depending on limitations such as money, support, organizational skills, family preferences, and home dynamics. One thing most of us will agree on is that it is difficult.

Food is a constant in our lives for our bodies to live, grow and thrive. Yet, there are many perceptions, likes, dislikes, and cultural norms attached to food. Throw in a mixture of a growing family, unsupportive partners or roommates, steeped gender roles, and extended family preferences, and meal prepping becomes a never-ending source of pain, unfortunately. Let's take a walk down my memory lane and tease apart some experiences.

As a child, I was lucky to grow up in a suburb where fresh produce was available prior to the explosion of processed foods. There were some processed foods, but they likely didn't factor too much in our lives as they were either too expensive or not preferred by our amazing chef, my mother. I grew up with a staple of vegetarian "thali," aka a plate of veggies, bread, daal, rice, and condiments. Evenings would be light but generally healthy meals. The "evening treats" were far in between. Perfectionism in cooking has always been a thing of lengthy discussions and expectations, with women trying to achieve these impossible tasks of cooking perfectly to everyone's liking, with some rigid thinking being passed down. "Food can only be cooked this way because when I didn't have any power, someone with more power in my household foisted their choices on us and got adored for it" or other similar rigidity and cycle of abuse.

As teenagers, we started hearing things about meat being better for your health, or some cricketer who was a lifelong vegetarian was forced to change to a meat-based diet as he couldn't bowl as far with just a poor vegetarian diet. A friend once told me that her brother had to start eating meat as that was considered healthy in the United States, where he had moved. More such stories came from friends/family about adopting Western culture in food as well. Slowly, fast foods and meat-heavy meals became quite popular in India. Somehow, I could never fathom making the change myself, as I had grown up eating a vegetarian healthy diet that had served me well. Also, I could not figure out why living healthily now necessitated everyone to start eating animal meat. I didn't bother to find out more at that time, as ethically, I knew I would remain vegetarian.

When I moved to the USA for my MPH, the food options were quite limited without having a car to drive around. Generally, you could find some oily or high-calorie options like pizza or Chinese foods. I learned to cook for myself, time permitting in between my studies, work, medical board exams (USMLE) prep, etc. As a result, my weight crept up quite a bit. Then, the deceptive logic of "a calorie is a calorie," regardless of the source of the food, became widespread, and I stumbled across it. Nutrition education in my medical school in India was limited to Preventive and Social Medicine which also used this faulty logic of measuring calories. So, sitting in the US, I secretly wanted to believe that a 100-calorie Twinkie is just that, a 100-calorie snack. Despite these measures, my weight kept creeping up—partly because I was barely sleeping, trying to do it all in a 24-hour day. I was introduced by a friend to the concept of "protein" in your diet and the paradoxical question, "Where do you get your protein?" Now in hindsight and thanks to apps like Chronometer, I can easily say, "It is everywhere in my plant-based diet," but then I did not know a good comeback when I needed one, that "Vegetarian food is just fine, thank you."

Rigorous medical residency was not the best time to make changes, although, in fellowship, I did start working out more and taking better care of my health through my first pregnancy. After having my children, I wanted to regain my health and fitness. During maternity leave, I read up on traditional Indian methods of post-pregnancy care and followed them to the extent possible. One advantage was working with my yoga teacher, Mrs. More, while she helped coach me back to health postpartum.

To better help my growing children, I took a step back, switched to a part-time schedule, and focused on all of our health. One day, I was blessed to attend the "Plants for Life" class with Dr. Steven Lawenda's team. The information was revolutionary. One message was that you can eat according to your own sensibilities and become healthier, and maintain your health. It laid the foundation in my mind and started the seeds which lead to Lifestyle Medicine (LM).

These changes were initially tough to wrap my mind around. Here is where the magic of social support comes in; one of our friend groups started a plant-based challenge a year later. (Thank you, Sadhana and Radhika!) Given it was just for three weeks, I thought, "Well, why not?" My husband, Mayank, and I made the switch to oat milk, stopped milk-based desserts completely, but most importantly, started incorporating high amounts of fiber in our diets. Three weeks went by quickly, and we were already feeling a change in our stamina and sleep. Then suddenly, the COVID-19 pandemic lockdowns began. I decided to continue the momentum, as working remotely gave us a chance to prepare our lunches differently. Six months later, we were looking younger than in our wedding pictures and also feeling lighter, with greater stamina for family walks and bike rides over the summer. I can only begin to express my gratitude for all of my mentors on the way, be it the friends I mentioned, countless plant-based cooking videos on YouTube, or excellent books by many authors such as Dr. Greger and Dr. Barnard. Thanks to the efforts of Dr. Pankaj Vij and his team, many of us interested doctors were able to take the Lifestyle Medicine boards in 2020 and get certified.

You may be wondering why you should get certified in LM. Each one of us will give you a different enthusiastic answer. Some physicians like LM for offering an alternative to just prescribing medications to their patients. Others have their own personal health journey to share. Most of us will agree that in Lifestyle Medicine, you find a community of "can-do" folks. For a long time, we have been taught to think that we cannot do anything to help our health. We have been falsely led to believe that any changes in the status quo will not only be unsuccessful but also lead to worsening health issues. But I'm here, and all of us are here to tell you differently.

Why is Lifestyle Medicine a good fit for me?

"If both of your parents have hypertension/diabetes mellitus type 2, there is a 45% probability for you to get the same diseases." I remember learning this in Preventive and Social Medicine in medical school in India. Also, growing up, I saw my grandmother use injectable insulin (the older vial form) on a daily basis and still deteriorate in health rapidly. Unfortunately, she developed gangrene, non-alcoholic fatty liver disease (NAFLD), and had a difficult end of life. Both my parents were diagnosed with diabetes mellitus (DM) type 2 and hypertension (HTN) in their 40s/50s. My father, being a physician, took great care of both of them and used state-of-the-art approaches available then medically (1990s era). They are still suffering from these issues today. My mother has since then gone on to have end-stage renal disease and has been on hemodialysis. How I wish we had access to the wonders of a whole food plant-based, evidence-based approach prior to these incidents! Many families like ours would have different experiences, being able to live, travel and prosper rather than being stuck in hospitals every other day.

My personal struggles came in the form of hyperinsulinemia after crossing age 35. I would feel like passing out after lunch, forget completing my workday, and doing all the chores pending at home. I stumbled upon Eastern wisdom, and some influencers like Dr. Jagannath Dixit understood we needed to take a closer look at diagnosing insulin resistance early on, not waiting for it to turn into full-blown diabetes mellitus type 2. When I made that mindset shift of beating insulin resistance, I could take ownership and change the trajectory of my health and wellness quite thoroughly.

Why did we write this book now?

To empower others to take charge of their health destiny.

I have traveled to India several times recently, and I see the same tropes repeating in the developing world that the West has seen for decades. Opinions that there are "right and wrong proteins" and only ingesting foods that will give a food corporate entity profit can be considered healthy. At the same time, I see the other side—women being burdened with cooking with the "just right," meaning excessive amounts of ghee and oil, on cooking shows and in real life, to prove their worth as mothers, wives, daughters, without a care to their own health long term. I see rigid "set points" of how each meal should feel extremely luxurious to pacify our feelings instead of true coping skills. Unfortunately, this kind of scenario is also worsening disordered eating and chronic health issues the world over.

How can Lifestyle Medicine help?

It helps by knowing what is evidence-based. It can be adapted to your cultural tastes and still carry your values. You can make small changes or moderate changes. We, LM doctors, are looking at the whole picture, from the importance of social connections and sleep to taking the reins and responsibility for our health in our own hands up to the greatest extent possible.

<u>Why social connection?</u>

Imagine you are a working mother who has no one sharing the mental labor of meal planning, leave alone letting her eat food the way she likes. It does not happen. Many people I see in my practice are stuck in these silos. Social connection brings you validation and stress relief and helps you with your communication skills. You come closer to understanding what your innermost needs around food, security, and health even are. We all need a "Find My Tribe" project.

There are many benefits of rethinking and reworking even the smallest aspects of our lives. Like James Clear emphasizes in his book _Atomic Habits_, even small changes over time will accrue to a more fulfilling life.

This book is the secret sauce on _How Healers Heal,_ and you can too. Yes, it seems daunting, and there are ways to overcome challenges.

<u>Steps to Simple Changes:</u>

1. Figure out which method works for you—whether setting a three-week challenge or slowly cutting back over time—there are no right or wrongs, just work with your strengths. The three-week challenge worked for me as there was a group of us motivating each other. Gradual changes work in an easier manner if food security is an issue or simply, your time is too overscheduled at the moment to do it otherwise.

2. Keep reading more recipes, listening to blogs, and getting in-spired for a whole food plant-based diet. What you read, hear, and see, you end up actually cooking and eating. Your taste buds

will evolve over time.

3. Take baby steps. Buy ingredients for one salad, a few soups, and some bean cans to begin. It's the worst feeling to have to throw away groceries from the fridge that you didn't get the time to cook.

4. Enlist help from family, you should NOT be doing it all. Limit the number of things cooked per meal in your household. Too many people try to have 2–3 different menus as they are internalizing other folks' misguided expectations. If teenagers or grown adults want a different meal, they can step into the kitchen and fix themselves a sandwich or some similar food.

5. Prep or plan for the week with your significant other if possible. Share ideas the week before, not when everyone is in HALT—Hungry, Angry, Lonely, or Tired.

6. It is okay to step away or take a break; health, work, and other issues happen in life. Flexibility, not rigidity, is our aim.

7. Have utmost compassion for any and all efforts that you make.

8. Sleep: Drawing boundaries and getting help with kitchen and chores . . . leads you to have time to do other things, including catching up on your sleep. Use a tracker or a simple sleep diary.

9. Exercise: Move a little bit every day. Don't wait for the best day to move; it doesn't show up for us regular folks. Take up hiking, gardening, or other outdoor activities away from screens.

10. Social connections, meditation, and spirituality: The glue that binds all the other steps together. Find what works for you.

11. Enjoy! This is an amazing journey to begin self-discovery.

So next time someone asks you, "Where do you get your protein?" What do you think you will say?

———◆○◆———

Thank you for picking up this book, either out of curiosity or compulsion. The pages of our book hope to lend strength and inspire you to choose your health in the coming weeks.

Many thanks to my children, my parents, my sister, and my in-laws. My husband Mayank, thank you for striking the delicate balance of feedback and cheer to help navigate the myriad projects my brain dreams up.

I am grateful and privileged to have learned from the exemplary women physicians in Lifestyle Medicine, who continue to nurture me to climb new heights. (Yes, you know who you are).

———◆○◆———

References:

Clear, J. (2018b). *Atomic Habits*. Random House.

About Dr. Mitika Kanabar MD, MPH, FASAM, DipABLM

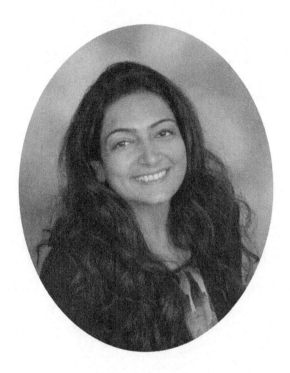

Dr. Mitika Kanabar completed her fellowship in Addiction Medicine at the prestigious Stanford University. She is triple board certified in Addiction Medicine, Lifestyle Medicine, and Family Medicine. Dr. Kanabar is dedicated to improving the lives of people with addictions and providing holistic care in recovery. She currently practices Addiction Medicine and Lifestyle Medicine in Southern California. Dr. Kanabar is an international public speaker on various addiction topics, including alcohol use, opioid use, gaming, digital overuse, and aspects of our relationship with food. Being motivated by yoga philosophy, Dr. Kanabar is an avid gardener and proponent of leading a balanced lifestyle.

Website: https://mitikakanabar.com/about-dr-mitika-kanabar/

Watch an interview with the co-author:

DR. MITIKA KANABAR

Scan Me

13

TWICE TRANSFORMED BY LIFESTYLE MEDICINE – AND STILL LEARNING

Mary Anne Kiel, MD, DipABLM, Col, USAF, MC

(The views expressed are those of the author and do not reflect the official views of the United States Air Force, nor the Department of Defense. Mention of trade names, commercial products, or organizations do not imply endorsement by the U.S. Government.)

"In our personal and professional lives, we are constantly hit with one adversity after the other, most of which we have no control over. But the four things we have total control over is how we react, how we adapt, how we breathe, and how we take action."

— Diamond Dallas Page

"What is your biggest life goal right now? What do you want most out of your future?"

My new fitness coach's voice was confident and clear over the computer, yet welcoming and curious too. She said she wanted to get to know me better first and asked me a series of questions, which I did my best to answer one by one.

I responded, "I want to feel better. I want to have energy. I want to be able to do the things I want to do and be an engaged mom while accomplishing what I need to at work."

She continued to ask me probing questions, which I answered matter-of-factly without letting on my frustration with how chaotic my life was.

"My job? I'm a pediatrician for the military. I take care of the service members' children. And I'm also our pediatric department head for both inpatient and outpatient care at our hospital.

"My hours? I work between 65–75 hours per week. I work mostly daytime hours, but every week I do at least one 36-hour overnight on-call shift. Once a month I cover a full week (including a weekend) of on-call and inpatient care. This can sometimes lead to staying awake for long periods of time over several days."

"My family? I am a wife and mother of three, ages 16, 11, and 6. My husband helps a lot—we both stay busy with the kids and work full time."

I was feeling so overwhelmed and busy every second of the day. I needed to figure out how to make time to exercise. I thought that would be helpful for so many of my issues: being overweight, chronic fatigue (falling asleep within one minute any time I sat in a semi-reclined position), and high cholesterol, which I'd had since my early 20s when I joined the military. At that time, I was told that my cholesterol was high, likely related to my family history, but not high enough to treat with medications, so the plan was to "continue to monitor it." Throughout the years, I was retested and told other recommendations like "take fish oil," "eat a more balanced diet" (but I was never really told what that meant), and "maybe consider a statin medication someday if it gets any higher."

Who was this fitness coach asking all of these additional questions? I just wanted her to tell me how to make time for exercise!

She asked, "Who does the cooking and grocery shopping?"

"Mostly me. During the week, we each prepare our own breakfasts. Lunch is usually leftovers for me because if I don't bring lunch to work and eat at my desk while I work, I won't get to eat, and I won't get all of my work done. Dinner is eaten as a family—I typically cook (except when my husband barbeques 1–2 times a week). We only drink sodas about once a week. Same for alcohol. Snacks are mostly healthier options like fruits, yogurt, crackers, low-fat cheese sticks, peanut butter with fruit, and granola bars. Weekend breakfasts are more elaborate, with the usual eggs, bacon, and toast or pancakes. I do practically all of the grocery shopping about once every 1–2 weeks."
"Any history of smoking?" she asked. "None," I said.

"How about sleep?" she inquired.
"Sleep?" I asked.

Interesting that this fitness coach was asking me about my sleep . . . I had not expected this topic to come up.

"Well, I struggle with sleep because of my job responsibilities. On average, I get about 5 hours of sleep each night. On weekdays, I work a full day (about 12 hours), come home, cook dinner, spend time with family, and get the kids to bed. Then, I often work another 1–3 hours on my laptop, finishing patient charts or other administrative tasks. Sometimes I work from home, but other times I either stay late at the office or go back in to get my work done because the computer network is faster. About once a week, I also do an overnight call shift (after working a full day) where sleep can be frequently interrupted and often no sleep.

Sometimes I get to leave work early the next afternoon to go home to sleep. I'm always sleepy . . ."

To be honest, I was hating my job. I felt like a hamster on a wheel—always with a pile of work that I couldn't get through, starting my day with a laundry list of items that I knew would never get crossed off, waking in the night with my mind racing about things I had forgotten to do or with heart palpitations about the day ahead. I felt trapped. There were times that I would take a day of leave just to play catch up on administrative work. I resented the fact that I was always at the hospital, but I didn't see a way to make it better.

My coach's inquisitive voice snapped me back to attention. "How about physical activity? You may not have much time for that, but what have you tried in the past? What types of exercise do you like doing? Are you doing any specific activity currently?"

I felt guilty in my response: "It's true that I'm not doing much activity currently. That's why I've set up this meeting with you. My goal is to make time for routine exercise. It's hard for me to feel motivated when my life is so chaotic. I'm gearing up for my military physical fitness test in about six months, and I'd love to do very well on it. I mostly enjoy aerobics, not so much the running or weightlifting, but I've got to get my run time down to pass my fitness test."

My coach said she wanted to have a better idea about the foods I ate, so she asked me to keep a food log of everything I ate and drank for a couple of days. Then she said: "First, I'd like to suggest that we work together on sleep."

What? That's interesting . . . I never thought my fitness coach would be coaching me about *sleep*. I wasn't sure at the time that my sleep was going to get any better with my hectic schedule. I know better now, but then I was surprised that she was suggesting I tackle sleep first before launching into a workout routine.

That's how it started—my first step on this new journey, which began seven years ago. My fitness coach and I continued to meet and talk "virtually" over the next two years (I was in Nevada, and she was in Florida, well before "virtual" was such a popular thing to do). She helped me control what I could with my sleep schedule, understanding that there would be things I couldn't control . . . especially with my work situation. On nights when I wasn't on call, she helped me make a bedtime routine. She banned my laptop from the bedroom and discouraged me from staying up late to finish work from home or after the duty day. It was really challenging at first, but I learned to prioritize what needed to be completed during the day, saving some of the work for my on-call days. However, it was a gamble, as sometimes the on-call work prevented me from having any spare time to complete the administrative work. I also learned to do a better job delegating tasks—to my husband, my kids, and my colleagues . . . this was definitely not in my nature. I had spent decades trying to "do it all" but failing miserably.

Her coaching absolutely helped, but ultimately, it took a bold career change to get a better handle on my sleep with a new job that had more administrative responsibilities but no nighttime calls and rare weekends. It was only then that I realized how important sleep was to my body and my brain . . . and my family. I was literally a ghost to them before, only halfway in the conversation, usually plotting how I could get in a few minutes of sleep without them noticing . . . maybe during an afternoon movie or while the kids were next door playing with their friends. I felt like what I imagined someone suffering from substance abuse might feel—always craving, never getting enough, seeking, feeling guilty, hiding my "using," cranky, and angry when I didn't get enough. All of us physicians, and especially me, always boasted that we could get by on such little sleep like it was a superpower. And I was blind to it . . . I couldn't accept how my lack of sleep was affecting me and those around me. It wasn't until I'd had 7–8 hours of consistent sleep every night for two years that I was able to see the difference . . . until I didn't fall asleep while sitting on the couch—when my kids finally stopped joking about "mom's falling asleep again during the movie!"—or feel the need to take a mid-afternoon nap . . . and when my husband seemed happier that I was able to engage in conversation and stay awake for some intimate time together.

About a year into my fitness coaching, my husband came across an article in the newspaper about a man who had successfully lost weight and reversed his chronic diseases by eating a whole food plant-based diet (WFPBD). My husband had been suffering from his own health concerns: overweight, sleep apnea requiring a CPAP machine at night, high blood pressure, and high cholesterol. He had not been following me on my fitness journey, so I was particularly surprised when he showed interest in this nutrition article, suggesting we should try it out.

At the time, I thought our diets were pretty good. We only ate out about once a week, although my husband ate out for lunch most days, and when we did eat out as a family, it was often from fast food locations like burger joints or chain restaurants. I didn't think we bought too many processed meals or foods, but looking back on it now, our pantry was full of cereals, crackers, chips, and cookies. We minimized sodas and juice (except for orange juice on weekends), drank low-fat milk, used margarine, and tried to stick with leaner cuts of meat. As a pediatrician, I thought I recognized the importance of nutrition even though I had never had any formal training. I tried to keep our meals "balanced" with a vegetable, a starch, and a lean meat or fish. I made sure my kids got their daily recommended servings of dairy (now we've switched to healthier plant-based options). I was skeptical of this WFPBD, which was something I had never heard of. But my husband was interested in learning more, so I agreed.

Over the next month, I read many articles about WFPBD. Much of the information was completely new to me, such as how animal products were contributing to chronic diseases, like my husband's high blood pressure and my high cholesterol. I was surprised to hear about the negative effects of dairy. I was familiar with how processed foods contributed to some chronic diseases, but I did not realize that even the processed foods we had in our pantry and freezer (the ones I thought were healthier options) were detrimental to our health (like the Goldfish crackers my kids loved and the egg white turkey sausage breakfast sandwiches I had bought for when I ran out the door late for work in the mornings). Even being a pediatrician who was health conscious, I was truly astonished at the dietary overhaul that was going to be expected of us with this whole food plant-based approach.

I recall my husband and I having many discussions about whether we could do this. What would life be like without eating processed foods and animal products? We suddenly realized that eggs, meat, and dairy were in every one of our meals. How would we do it? What would we eat? How would it feel when we went out to eat or over to friends' houses or on holidays? It seemed like such a bizarre concept to us, but the health impacts we were reading about propelled us to give it a try.

We started almost immediately. We had no idea what we were doing. We laugh, looking back on it now. It was not very fun in the beginning, as I either burned a lot of food or had mushy, tasteless food. I quickly realized that I needed help. I did some searching and came upon an online cooking class called Rouxbe: Plant-Based Cooking Course. Although I was terribly busy in my former job as a pediatrician and department chief, I knew I had to make this a priority if we were going to have any chance at success. On nights and weekends when I wasn't taking calls at the hospital, my husband and I worked through the online recipes and cooked the meals. We learned new skills that laid the foundation for how we cook today: how to chop, dry sauté, and roast without oil. It was actually fun to have a new project as a couple. And even amid a very busy three-month period (a temporary duty assignment for me involving a week of military field training, the end of the kids' school year, and my new job, which took our family to a new home in a new state across the country), we still managed to complete the assignments for the cooking school. We felt tremendously satisfied and successful! It was still all new to us, trying to navigate the recipes and cooking techniques, but at least we had some strategies to help.

It was not too long after that when I stumbled upon a health conference advertisement called the <u>Plantrician Project</u>. I almost couldn't believe that there was a health professional conference about WFPBD! I was relieved to find other physicians looking into this too. Our new way of eating seemed very "fringe" . . . almost like quackery, and I remember feeling unsure and embarrassed to talk about it among colleagues for fear of them thinking I was too "radical." It felt like my family and I were the only ones in our little bubble doing this. I needed to hear what other health professionals were saying about the medical evidence. Despite the cost and the time commitment away from work, I purchased the registration and got ready for San Diego.

The Plantrician Project medical conference blew my mind! I recall sitting through a presentation, listening to Dr. Anthony Lim's talk about calorie density and how type 2 diabetes can be reversed through eating a whole food plant-based diet . . . unbelievable! I almost cried. After four years of medical school, three years of residency, and 12 years as a practicing pediatric staff physician, how is it possible I had never heard of this? I sat through so many incredible presentations during that conference and met a number of healthcare professionals and other individuals who were on a similar path—excited to improve their health and that of their patients by getting to the root causes of disease by applying the basics of what I came to learn was the field of Lifestyle Medicine: maximizing nutritious food, sleep, movement, positive social connections, managing stress and removing risky substances. I heard story after story of individuals having reversed disease by intensively applying these mechanisms when the maximal conventional medicine regimens had previously failed them. It was liberating, empowering, and almost too good to be true! I returned home with a new passion for what I was doing . . . like I had a secret that could change people's lives, including mine. I yearned to learn even more and to start putting some of it into practice.

After returning home, my inclination was to find out whether there were others in the Air Force practicing Lifestyle Medicine. I had never heard anything about it before in our Military Health System, but like any vast organization, staying fully aware of every resource can be challenging. I did a number of internet searches and stumbled upon a prior news article highlighting an Air Force pediatrician who had begun a Lifestyle Medicine program several years prior at Yokota Air Base, Japan. I recall tremendous excitement about finding a colleague in this same space, and we were soon able to connect for a phone call. He had recently separated from the military, but he put me in touch with several of his Air Force colleagues practicing Lifestyle Medicine. It was truly motivating to hear that a handful of others in my organization were passionate about this way of living and were working to promote it among their patients! I set out to make other connections with those individuals through a number of scheduled conference calls to learn from them and see how we could collaborate.

As I was starting to explore more about Lifestyle Medicine professionally, I was also on a new path to integrate more of it into my personal life. I read numerous articles, listened to podcasts, and watched documentaries. A new world had opened up to me, and I was jumping into it with both feet! I began swapping ingredients for our meals at home, removing the animal products and oils, trying new recipes, and putting into practice what I had learned from various sources. My husband and I both saw dramatic health improvements over the course of the next six months: my cholesterol panel completely normalized (after having had borderline high levels for the past 20 years!), I lost 25 pounds without trying, and I had more energy and less brain fog. My husband lost 50 pounds, lost six inches of waist circumference, improved his cholesterol, and normalized his blood pressure (which had always been 130–150s/90–100s at his doctors' appointments, but he had never been on treatment because the clinicians always chalked it up to "white coat hypertension"). The most dramatic improvement was that his snoring improved so much that his repeat sleep study showed his sleep apnea had resolved, and he no longer needed his CPAP machine! This was a huge accomplishment for my husband, and he was thrilled not to have to lug that machine around when he traveled!

My children, however, were a little less enthused. They had grown up with our former way of eating and were struggling somewhat to embrace this new approach. At this point, they were in their teen years/young adulthood. We did our best to stick to familiar meals they could still appreciate by just swapping in plant-based items for animal products, but it obviously wasn't an equivalent taste. They were strongly set on their food preferences based on what they previously ate. We allowed them autonomy to pick whatever they wanted when we ate out at restaurants (although admittedly, the restaurant options were new and somewhat limited since my husband and I were being much more selective about which ones we ate at—no more fast-food dives or chains!).

We continued to try. I studied more resources. I voraciously watched webinars and continuing education seminars. I was learning so much, and I felt like each new information morsel I soaked up was helping me turn my life around. I didn't realize it then, but I was channeling this extra energy and passion with my new additional free time, thereby essentially swapping my former sleep-deprived self with this overly consumed self. My mind was constantly spinning in a state of thought and planning, even when at the dinner table with family or while trying to enjoy an evening activity. I was either reading a lifestyle-related book, listening to a nutrition podcast, or studying the Lifestyle Medicine board exam material on my laptop. I became obsessed with soaking up as much of this new information as I could—to the point that it was almost all I talked about. It was definitely almost all I thought about! My conversation centered quite frequently on nutrition or things related to disease prevention. It wasn't apparent to me then, but I had simply traded my previous work-soaked life for a new priority which was commandeering my life and eroding my relationships. I would do my best to listen and pay attention to what my husband and children were talking about in conversation, but it seemed that my mind would almost instantly be derailed and switch to something else. My family grew frustrated after I unknowingly (but frequently) asked them questions or attempted to make conversation, only to stop listening part way through their responses . . . or when I would ask the same question again—even though they had just answered it a few moments before. I went so far as to have an audiology examination to make sure nothing was wrong with my hearing! I recall the audiologist gently telling me that the ears were just one part of the pathway required for hearing and that, many times, it was the mind that needed to be tamed.

It was later that year when I had some unexpectedly devastating news. My husband of 20 years asked me for a divorce. It was particularly traumatic for me because I had not expected it at all—I was blindsided. I was trying so hard to do everything right, and I felt like I had made so much progress personally with my sleep issues, stress management, professional career, personal health, and so on. However, despite my positive changes, what I came to realize over the next two years was that I still had much to learn and practice about being present in the moment, developing mindfulness, and cultivating my relationships. My husband was hurting and lonely, but I hadn't realized it. He was adamant about separating. I insisted on counseling to help us prepare to co-parent, which he obliged. A lot came out during those sessions—things we had never discussed . . . tears from both of us . . . some anger and fear, truth, and hesitation. Each of us learned new skills. Feeling unsure about letting a stranger into our deepest thoughts and relationship . . . but learning to trust the therapist and each other over time. It has taken a long time and lots of work for both of us, but we recommitted ourselves to our relationship as a married couple. We're by no means perfect, but I believe we learned a lot about our own selves and each other through this experience. We are in a better place now.

In the midst of our relationship discord, I explored ways to help tame my mind. I had never practiced meditation before. In fact, I had never had much quiet time before . . . always on the go (if not sleeping!). When

I was not physically moving, I was mentally moving: planning, making lists, and checking emails. Never an idle moment. Even while watching a movie with my family, I would spend the time folding laundry, doing dishes, or other tasks often involving my laptop. Meditation was hard at first. Every fiber in my body revolted against it. My brain could focus on two breaths at most, and then it was off tackling what I was going to prepare for dinner. I would yank it back to attention like it was on a leash. Oh right, I was supposed to "gently bring my mind back to focus on the breath." It took significant practice. Five minutes here and there throughout the week was, at times, all I could muster. Once, I managed to meditate daily for three weeks straight, which was my longest streak. Even though I didn't always practice it daily, I did notice that my mind's ability to attend to the matter at hand was significantly better after several months. When I had spinning thoughts, a racing mind, or stress, I was able to recognize it quickly and make time for meditation and calm. My therapist helped me understand that my presence (not just my physical presence, but my mental presence too), even when it was just watching a movie, was important to my family, especially my husband. I worked on sitting "idle" and being present during these activities. This was extremely hard for me, as I had not done this in decades. Over time, it became easier, and my family seemed to appreciate it.

These days, my life is, thankfully, a bit slower-paced. Professionally, I am intimately involved in integrating Lifestyle Medicine into the Military Health System. Our small group of like-minded healthcare professionals has grown to a formally recognized Air Force Lifestyle & Performance Medicine Working Group with several hundred members from across all the military services. We are sharing the benefits of Lifestyle Medicine with our staff and active duty service members. Lifestyle Medicine has brought back my passion for medicine. Although what our working group has accomplished thus far fills me with pride, I am even more grateful for what Lifestyle Medicine has done for me in my personal life. It has given me and my family our health back. It has changed my perspective in immeasurable ways. I like to think I am a better wife and mom, a better friend, and a better human because of Lifestyle Medicine.

———◆◇◆———

This chapter is to my Husband and Children: thank you for not giving up on me!

And to my former Self: in celebration to acknowledge how strong, brave, and dedicated you were despite the many challenges and how far you've come with learning new skills!

And to my future Self: may you continue to grow, remain curious, and look back with joy on a life well-lived!

———◆◇◆———

References:

Girard, J., & Thomas, D. (Directors). *Rouxbe Online Culinary School*. Rouxbe. https://rouxbe.com/.

The Plantrician Project (501c3 not-for-profit corporation). The Plantrician Project: Planting the Seeds of Change. https://plantricianproject. org/.

About Dr. Mary Anne Kiel, MD, DipABLM, Col, USAF, MC

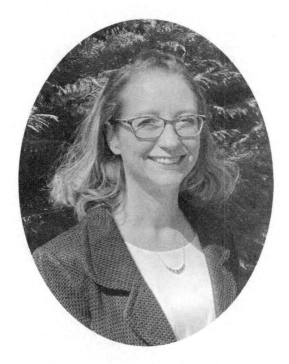

As of the writing of this book, Dr. Mary Anne Kiel is a Colonel and Pediatrician in the United States Air Force who is board certified in both Pediatrics and Lifestyle Medicine. She is stationed at the Defense Health Headquarters in Falls Church, Virginia, where she leads the Air Force Medical Home program and the Air Force Lifestyle & Performance Medicine Working Group. She and her husband lead a plant-based lifestyle and enjoy capturing medals for their virtual walking challenges, playing board games, and traveling. They are the proud parents of their three children and puppy dog, Oscar. Dr. Kiel is passionate about helping her family members, her patients, and active duty service members live their best lives by practicing the pillars of Lifestyle Medicine.

LinkedIn: https://www.linkedin.com/in/mary-anne-kiel-3b1b90132

Watch an interview with the co-author:

DR. MARY ANNE KIEL

Scan Me

14

Our Genes Do Not Determine Our Destiny: A Palliative Care Doctor and BRCA1 Previvor's Journey to Embracing Lifestyle and Mindset

Simran Malhotra, MD, DipABLM, CHWC

"Sometimes the bad things that happen in our lives put us directly on the path to the best things that will ever happen to us."

— Unknown

Cancer and I crossed paths for the first time when I was only 13 years old when my mom was diagnosed with breast cancer at the young age of 33 years old. Since then, I have had many life-altering experiences—my own, those of the people closest to me, and even the stories shared by many of my seriously ill patients—some of whom shared two things in common with me, a genetic mutation, cancer, *or both.*

Eight years ago, in 2015, I was 27 years old, finishing up residency, and getting ready to tie the knot with the love of my life when I got my genetic test results back showing that I carried the breast cancer 1 (BRCA1) genetic mutation —the same mutation I had read about in medical school that could now magnify my lifetime breast cancer risk by up to 87% and ovarian cancer by 50–60%. I remember sitting in the genetic counselor's office with my fiancée when she shared the results of my pathogenic BRCA1 gene. Tears streamed down our cheeks as we held hands tightly, both of us feeling a rush of emotions at that moment. We were all too familiar with what cancer looks like up close, which left us feeling overwhelmed with all that may lie ahead.

A year prior, my mom had discovered that she carried a pathogenic variant of BRCA1 after I encouraged her to retest many years after her initial diagnosis and following the news of another close family member who had been recently diagnosed with primary peritoneal carcinoma (an aggressive and rare form of ovarian cancer). This diagnosis was the red flag that sounded the alarm for me that something in my family was _not right_. From there, I began digging into my maternal history, which was hard since discussing cancer, illness, and death is just not what we do in my family, nor is it part of the cultural South Asian norm. Yet I persisted, and what I found was shocking. Sadly, nine women in my family (to date) have experienced some form of breast or ovarian cancer—my mom is a two-time breast cancer survivor and thriver today. A number of these courageous souls are no longer with us here Earthside.

The year I found out about my mutation was the year I also started my specialty training in hospice and palliative care—a field specializing in caring for people living with serious life-threatening illnesses, often nearing the end of their physical life. This was an especially challenging time as I tried to navigate understanding what my genetic mutation meant for me and my future while also caring for several young patients with advanced cancers. I began to see up close what cancer can take away from a patient and a family, but also what resilience and hope looked like. There was one young woman in her 40s with advanced ovarian cancer, who happened to carry the same genetic mutation as me, who changed my life. A few days before she died, she found out I carried the same mutation as she did and said, "Simran, don't let this happen to you. Do whatever you need to do to live a full life and stay alive for your future children. You have a choice." In that instant, she lit the flame of curiosity, knowledge, and power in my heart. I learned how to use that fire to make informed decisions about my life and learned not to take no for an answer. This was exactly the sense of control I needed when everything around me seemed chaotic and uncertain. At that time, I didn't know exactly what that meant for me, but I vowed to find out.

The next steps became clear as I met with a medical team made up of genetic counselors, oncologists, breast surgeons, plastic surgeons, etc., who all shared with me the latest data on risk reduction in women carrying a BRCA1 mutation, particularly with my strong family penetrance which included serial imaging and surveillance, as well as prophylactic surgeries once I was done childbearing. So here I was, 27 years old, and I had five very big life milestones that needed to be accomplished within the next six years. One of them was prophylactic surgeries, per my medical team, by the age of 33—the same age my mom was first diagnosed with breast cancer.

And they went as follows:

Number 1: Finish my fellowship training, take two board exams, and start my mandatory three-year visa commitment as a full-time palliative care physician. (Ah, the joys of being on a visa as a Canadian!)

Number 2: Marry my best friend.

Number 3: Schedule my biannual surveillance, which included a clinical breast exam, mammograms, and MRIs (which went on to become a series of unexpected poking and prodding of my breasts to biopsy areas that were considered suspicious due to my family history. Let me tell you, this was not fun!).

Number 4: Get pregnant, have children, and be sure I was done having children.

Number 5: Get my prophylactic risk-reducing surgeries.

If you're thinking, wow, that is a lot—well, that is exactly how I felt most days. The number of emotions and challenges I faced during those years almost felt like too much to bear at times. Fear, anxiety, and heartache deepened every time I cared for a young woman with advanced cancer, which only worsened if she had kids, as I found out in early 2016 that my husband and I were expecting our first child. Even though this was the most wonderful event which had ever happened to us, it also made my already difficult days at work even more intimidating at times.

Fast-forward 1.5 years later to 2017, I took on two new full-time jobs: one as a newly minted palliative care physician and one as a new mother. I felt as though I was constantly having to juggle my work and personal life. From nursing to pumping to getting cancer screenings and navigating the psychological impacts of work while maintaining our home, these daily challenges tested my resilience more than ever before. We were emotionally and physically drained, yet so blessed to find out I was pregnant again when my daughter was only nine months old. Life was about to get even busier, but making the decision to have our kids back-to-back allowed me to breastfeed each of them for a year while still being able to get my preventative surgeries done before I turned 33 years old. During this period, there was practically no downtime! Despite the chaos, my patient's voice constantly reminded me that something needed to shift, not only for that moment but also for my future and the future of my family. And at that point, I still didn't really know what to expect on the road (or years) ahead.

Since the day I got my genetic test results, my medical team told me there was nothing else I could do aside from frequent high-risk screenings, medications, or surgeries to reduce my risk of cancer. Yet despite this and my constantly asking them the same questions, I knew there was something I could do because one of my core beliefs is:

There is always something that you can do.

During one sleepless night in early 2017, while nursing my baby, I stumbled upon a Google search that eventually led me to Dr. Michael Greger's work and research. What I discovered was simply mind-blowing. It ultimately changed the trajectory of my life in a moment!

The next day, a copy of his book *How Not to Die* arrived on my doorstep, and I dove right in. His book starts with the story of his 65-year-old grandmother suffering from end-stage heart disease who was ultimately sent home on hospice care—something I was all too familiar with as a palliative care physician. I was shocked by what I read next—that she managed to turn her heart disease around through intensive lifestyle changes and lived another 30 years until she passed away in her 90s. As a palliative care physician caring for patients suffering from advanced heart disease, I couldn't help but wonder why I had never heard of this concept before. So much so that I even read and reread the text to make sure what I was reading was correct! I have had the unfortunate but eye-opening privilege of witnessing what chronic illness and debility can take away from not only a person but also their family. My patients often experience unbearable emotional, spiritual, and physical symptoms such as pain, anxiety, difficulty breathing, and social isolation, not to mention the loss of their freedom and independence. I was filled with a rush of questions: "Why had I not heard about Lifestyle Medicine (LM) before? Why had I never heard about the science behind it and the tremendous possibilities it carries?" And then I wondered, "Even if these interventions did not reverse every patient's disease, could lifestyle modifications improve the quality of life for my patients?" After all, improving someone's quality of life was at the heart of everything I did in palliative care.

The numbers I came across were startling. According to the CDC, 60% of Americans have at least one chronic disease, while 40% have two or more. Half of all Americans have heart disease. Eighty-eight million Americans have prediabetes, yet 90% don't even know it. Today, one out of every four deaths is from cancer. The leading causes of death globally are mostly related to lifestyle habits, with a suboptimal diet being the #1 risk factor for death. More than 80% of chronic diseases are preventable with healthy lifestyle changes. As I started thinking about my patients living with serious life-threatening, often end-stage, diseases, I started to redefine the definition of a serious illness. High blood pressure or high cholesterol may appear to be harmless, however, these conditions are the very first signs of common serious illnesses—also referred to as 'silent killers.' Often individuals live with these diseases for years while taking medications without addressing the root cause. Ultimately, these diseases lead to end-stage diseases, and patients have to consult a doctor like me. And it often isn't the patients seeking me out, but rather the medical team, as the medications and procedures are no longer able to slow down the progression of the patient's disease burden. Using lifestyle as medicine is something most conventionally trained physicians like me are not trained to emphasize. The most powerful realization I had, after becoming the patient myself, was that using modalities that empower and educate people on their diet, movement, social connectedness, and management of stress are all ways to not only give them back control of their lives but also to help them live longer, more meaningful lives.

In 2015, after I got married, I decided I was going to go from a standard Asian American diet to a vegetarian style of eating—at that time, it was for no reason other than there was way too much meat served at our wedding, and I simply needed a break. And then, after all I had learned after reading Dr. Greger's book and a few others, I transitioned to a mostly plant-based diet and ultimately, a plant-based vegan diet in 2018. I often get asked why? The answer is simple. Based on my research, a plant-predominant diet is going to be the best way to reduce my risk of cancer (along with reducing my risk of all the other top killers in America). The most beautiful part of my lifestyle changes has been watching the ripple effect on my husband, my family, and my friends.

I have seen incredible improvements in their blood pressure, cholesterol, constipation, energy levels, and weight loss. Many of them achieved outcomes they were not even TRYING to achieve but did so simply by increasing the consumption of plants in their diet, and that, my friend, is the power of plants!

By January 2020, I had just finished nursing my second baby. For the last three years, I had been in awe of the awesomeness of my breasts. I mean, they fed and grew two little humans for almost their entire first year of life. Then the realization suddenly hit me that my breasts could now be the reason why I don't get to witness them growing up.

Therefore, it was time for me to take action—it was time for surgery.

I braced myself to face surgery in the coming months and consulted with breast and plastic surgeons about the many options surrounding a preventative mastectomy and hysterectomy. The anxiety came flooding back, especially since I had been in the middle of caring for a young woman with advanced-stage cancer, diagnosed six months earlier, just a few weeks after having her baby. This experience made me want to get the surgery sooner than later. Yet the choices were daunting, and the multiple doctors' visits were exhausting. Should I get reconstruction with implants or get a flap? Or since I was small-breasted, to begin with, maybe I should just go flat? This latter option was not well supported by my initial team of doctors. Should I have a total hysterectomy now and throw myself into premature menopause at the age of 32, considering the youngest ovarian cancer diagnosed was at 31 years old in my mom's relative? Or maybe just take one ovary out, or maybe a salpingectomy (fallopian tube excision) should be good enough for now? As I was reflecting on all these thoughts, an unanticipated intruder shook up our lives—a global pandemic, the COVID-19 pandemic.

Life as we knew it changed. All outpatient and elective procedures were canceled, including my upcoming surgeries in June 2020. My husband, a critical care physician, moved into the basement, not knowing what we were up against. He was consumed in the trenches of caring for COVID patients in the intensive care unit (ICU). Suddenly our young children were not being tucked in at night by their dad and no longer going to school. I found myself knee-deep in virtual meetings with families whose loved ones were dying of severe COVID-related illnesses. Between the two of us, we saw more trauma, suffering, and death than we could have imagined—BRCA1 and surgeries became the last thing on my mind during those terrifying first few months.

On September 2, 2020, my husband dropped me off at the curbside of the hospital at 5:30 am, and I walked in alone to have a bilateral nipple-sparing mastectomy with aesthetic flat closure and a total hysterectomy putting me into surgical menopause at 32 years old . . . Phew! Unfortunately, I had a bleeding complication that landed me emergently on the trauma operating room (OR) table early the next morning. The only upside was that the hospital made an exception for my husband to be at my bedside after I got out of surgery. For the next several weeks, I needed assistance from my husband, mom, and friends for even my most basic needs, like using the bathroom and washing my hair. This was a pivotal moment in my life. Living a life of dependence, even for a few short weeks, showed me exactly what I didn't want my life to look like—in pain, dependent on others for care, and unable to care for myself. This was my call to action. For the first time in my life, I decided I was committing to my self-care or rather my self-preservation and quality of life. After eight weeks of healing, my doctors gave me the green light to start exercising again, and I haven't stopped since. It was the weeks after my surgery that ultimately prompted a total transformation of not just my lifestyle but, perhaps even more importantly, my mindset.

So today, I am 35 years old, with two young children, a palliative care physician married to a critical care physician, having recently served our sickest patients during the worst global pandemic of our time while having had multiple major surgeries, and I can tell you without a doubt, I have never known a better version of myself. So, what does this version of me today know that the 27-year-old version of me did not yet realize?

What I realized was that the most amazing things, the biggest opportunities, and the life-defining moments that happen to us are often disguised as impossible situations that are happening for us, not to us. These impossible situations are simply opportunities for us to grow—gifts that push us to become the next evolution of ourselves—wiser, bolder, and more resilient.

These opportunities allow us to rewrite our story and also become the bridge that someone else will one day walk over, with a little bit less pain and fear because we showed them the infinite possibilities lying ahead of them.

So, I have had many life-altering experiences—my own, those of the people closest to me, and the stories of my incredibly brave patients—and here is what I learned:

1. Wellness starts with your mindset.

Even though I felt empowered by my genetic mutation and my choices, I couldn't shake off the fear and anxiety of the future until I experienced and learned from what the COVID-19 pandemic had in store for us. The COVID-19 pandemic opened my eyes to how quickly life can change our plans and reinforced the importance of being mindful of each day as it unfolds rather than living in what was or will be. Harnessing the power of making informed decisions is important, but perhaps even more important is focusing on what is in our control in any given situation and taking action to move forward, even if it is the tiniest step in the direction we want to go. Ultimately, this focus allows us to design a life we can fall in love with every day regardless of what adversities are thrown our way. I realize that while mutations like mine can bring significant challenges, they also offer unique perspectives on life and how we approach each day. With every challenge I faced, I tried to find strength in the ups and downs and turned them into opportunities for growth and self-empowerment.

Taking small but powerful actions consistently on the things that are in my control in each season of my life, particularly the everyday mundane actions I take toward energizing my body and soul, has allowed me to stand guard at the entrance of my mind. Now I understand that if I can control my mind, anything is possible. Take it from me, regardless of how challenging your situation is right now, as I learned from one of my greatest role models, Tony Robbins, that we must believe that life is always happening for us, not to us, even if we can't always understand how right away. We can rise above any situation because no one can take away our ability to choose what to focus on, what meaning we give to our circumstances, and what actions we will take next.

2. Food is medicine. Movement is medicine. Sleep is medicine. Your lifestyle is the most powerful medicine that has ever existed.

If, like me, you are among the 5–10% of people with a genetic predisposition to cancer or another illness, let Dr. Ornish's words be your daily mantra: "Genes are not our fate." Though the genes we are born with may be beyond our control, the switches which determine whether some genes are turned on or "express" themselves or not remain in our hands. This privilege is what I like to call *epigenetic power*! Undoubtedly, you have already guessed it—diet, exercise, and sleep are some of the major influencers of epigenetics.

I radically transformed my lifestyle after the surgeries. My routine now consists of waking up at 5:30 am most of the week, incorporating movement and meditation. I aim to get 7–8 hours of sleep each night, and I have surrounded myself with a tribe of people who love me and who I am blessed to love. I follow a plant-based way of eating. During this busy season of my life, as a working mama with young kids, I am mindful to extend myself grace and understand that my best is enough. I am determined never to let perfection be the enemy of my progress.

As both a palliative care physician, who has witnessed significant suffering and pain, as well as an individual who knows the struggles of being a patient firsthand, I have come to realize that despite many of the modern medical advances, there is no doubt that investing in healthy habits is the most impactful and beneficial gift you can give yourself, as well as your family.

3. Live with an abundance of gratitude over fear.

In times of tragedy, it is incredibly difficult to find what we are grateful for, but it is not only possible but also healing. Keep it simple and write it down. Find gratitude for being able to breathe easy, love your family, or simply wake up to live another day. This has been a practice that has brought me immense joy and peace.

Over the years, I have accumulated decades' worth of life experiences from my dying patients, and many of their last words continue to be a profound reminder to me: "I wish I had loved more," "I wish I spent more time with my family," "My biggest regret was not doing what truly made me happy." So today, let's simply be grateful we have the opportunity to love, learn, grow, and be alive today.

When we live with an attitude of gratitude, the lens through which we see our challenges and our world changes. We become more aware of the gift of a beating heart that we have been given instead of focusing on all that is going wrong in our lives or in the world. Fear can easily turn into gratitude when you think about it from an abundance point of view. Being human is hard at times, _and_ it is also beautiful. And another core belief of mine is: *"I (we) can do hard, beautiful things."*

The beauty of exploring lifestyle medicine for the first time as a physician is you are your own first patient. My BRCA1 mutation changed my life in many ways, but the greatest gift it gave me was allowing me to discover the powerful effects of evidence-based lifestyle medicine—*my life's ultimate purpose.* It took me from *cancer awareness to ACTION against cancer*, not only through the advances in medical therapy but more significantly through embracing lifestyle habits that empowered me to transform the way I think, eat, move, sleep, manage stress, and connect with others.

My story is one of strength and courage in the face of adversity. I hope that I inspired you to cultivate a lifestyle allowing you to reach your highest potential and make the most out of this life we have been gifted. After all, life is too short to suffer. So, if you consider it, I encourage you to take one action today: love more, sleep well, move more, stress less, eat more plants, and be present. I'll leave you with what the incredible Art Berg once said, "Wherever you are along your journey, just hang on because the impossible just takes a little bit longer."

Dedicated to my mom, the strongest & fiercest woman I know, as well as my kids and husband — who endlessly love & support me.

References:

Casaubon, J. T. (2022, September 19). *BRCA 1 and 2.* StatPearls - NCBI Bookshelf. https://www.ncbi.nlm.nih.gov/books/NBK470239/.

Chronic Diseases in America | CDC. https://www.cdc.gov/chronicdise ase/resources/infographic/chronic-diseases.htm.

Afshin, A., Sur, P. J., Fay, K., Cornaby, L., Ferrara, G., Salama, J. K., Mullany, E. C., Abate, K. H., Abbafati, C., Abebe, Z., Afarideh, M., Aggarwal, A., Agrawal, S., Akinyemiju, T., Alahdab, F., Bacha, U., Bachman, V. F., Badali, H., Badawi, A., . . . Murray, C. J. L. (2019). Health effects of dietary risks in 195 countries, 1990–2017: a systematic analysis for the Global Burden of Disease Study 2017. *The Lancet, 393*(10184), 1958–1972. https://doi.org/10.1016/s0140-6736(19)30041-8.

Ornish, D., MD, & Ornish, A. (2019). *Undo It!: How Simple Lifestyle Changes Can Reverse Most Chronic Diseases.* Ballantine Books.

Greger, M., MD, & Stone, G. (2016b). *How Not to Die: Discover the Foods Scientifically Proven to Prevent and Reverse Disease.* Pan Macmillan. https://nutritionfacts.org/.

About Dr. Simran Malhotra, MD, DipABLM, CHWC

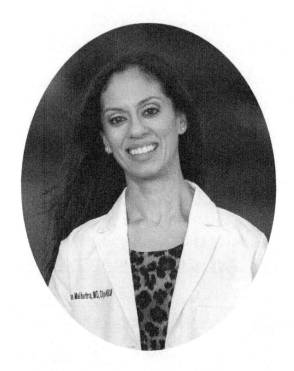

Dr. Simran Malhotra is a mother of two and a triple board-certified physician in Internal Medicine, Hospice and Palliative Care, and Lifestyle Medicine as well as a certified Health and Wellness Coach. In addition, she completed the T. Colin Campbell Plant-Based Nutrition Certification and the CHEF Culinary Coaching Certification. She has been featured on several blogs and podcasts where she has shared her unique perspectives and experiences from palliative care as well as from being a genetic mutation carrier who is passionate about using lifestyle as medicine. She founded Wellness by LifestyleMD, a platform where she educates women at high risk for cancer with or without genetic mutations on the powerful impact that positive lifestyle changes can have on their quality of life and longevity.

Website: http://www.wellnessbylifestylemd.com

Instagram: https://www.instagram.com/drsimran.malhotra/

LinkedIn: https://www.linkedin.com/in/simran-malhotra-md-66240110b/

Watch an interview with the co-author:

Co-Author spotlight
DR. SIMRAN MALHOTRA

Scan Me

15

Lifestyle Medicine – A Life Transformation

Erin Mayfield, DO, DipABLM, DipAOBOG

"He who has health has hope; and he who has hope, has everything."

— Thomas Carlyle

E mbracing Lifestyle Medicine (LM) and developing a new telemedicine practice at age 65 has been fun, challenging, rewarding, and disappointing. The practice of LM itself is thrilling, as it offers hope for the future health and longevity of all Americans. LM offers a total reversal of the health trends I have experienced practicing medicine for the past 39 years.

Personally, LM has helped me transform from a lifetime of overeating, weight gain, disinterest in cooking, fear of public speaking, and feeling uncomfortable in social situations. My journey has been liberating and FUN!

Professionally, LM educated me on up-to-date nutrition, fitness, and the science of behavior change. It required me to start a new medical practice. It motivated me to explore entrepreneurial opportunities in my new community and develop relationships that would benefit patients and their culinary medicine education. My professional activities since my personal adoption of LM include board certification in LM, certification as a Harvard Chef coach, teaching culinary medicine cooking classes to the general public, and multiple in-person and televised speaking engagements.

My introduction to LM began in the spring of 2019 when I discovered Lifestyle Medicine during my post-operative recovery from rotator cuff surgery. Backed by decades of evidence-based research and clinical application, LM demonstrates that physicians can successfully prevent and treat chronic diseases with lifestyle change. Prior to my discovery, I was already a whole food plant-based (WFPB) eater, having read Dr. T. Colin Campbell's book *The China Study* about seven years prior. Eliminating dairy and meat from my diet enabled me to cut cravings and lose 45 pounds naturally, using foods from the grocery store. I even started cooking! I had no idea at the time how LM would change my life. It was a dramatic transformation in so many ways and in a short period of time.

"We are not prisoners of our genetics. We have the power to change our destiny." – Dr. Erin Mayfield

As a gynecologist for over 30 years, I enjoyed seeing women for their annual preventative exams. Their visit was a wonderful opportunity to perform a thorough physical exam, review up-to-date health screening recommendations, and explore any problems that could be impacting their daily lives. The topics we discussed frequently mirrored the six lifestyle medicine pillars of health—nutrition, exercise, sleep, stress, relationships, and avoidance of cigarettes and alcohol.

Many of my gynecology patients struggled with the same types of problems year after year, including bleeding irregularities, weight gain, difficulty losing weight, difficulty sleeping, stress, and menopausal issues. We worked together as a team, drilling down to reveal the root cause of the problem; we created a reasonable plan of action to solve it. But many of my patients returned with the same issues, and it was a mystery to me as to why.

Completion of the LM board certification coursework updated me in nutrition science, the psychology of behavior change, modern coaching methods, sleep science, and exercise science. I finally understood why women gained weight easily and why it seemed impossible for women to lose weight—*because there was no ongoing support for behavior modification once they left my office. Behavior change is complex and challenging, especially when it involves culture and family.*

I was thrilled to be armed with these new coaching skills and for the potential to change my patients' lives. However, my husband and I had recently relocated to Florida, which meant starting a new medical practice. I contemplated the return on investment for my new education and the board certification exam fees. At the time, I was 63 years old. Most of my friends were retiring.

I visited the exam registration page for the American Board of Lifestyle Medicine (ABLM) multiple times. My change in jobs meant starting a medical practice in a new location where I had little community presence. Undeterred and moreover, with such passion for the work and excitement to participate in this movement, I studied and passed the LM exam in November 2019, the third class of diplomates of the ABLM!

Life in January 2020 presented new challenges as a global pandemic was brewing. By the spring of 2020, my new medical practice was launched as a telemedicine practice, structured to offer live interactive group coaching and live cooking classes via Zoom meetings. I maintained licensure in Florida and Georgia to serve as many people as possible. The most frustrating and time-consuming part of developing this new practice model was learning how to market it, and how to meet people in my new community and earn their trust. My new adventure threw me into the social media marketing world, a world that I knew nothing about.

I spent most of the pandemic year isolated at home, learning how to run my new business. By the end of the year, I had incorporated and named my new practice: Lifestyle Medicine Wellness and Recovery, LLC. The next steps for growth and reaching more patients included hiring a website developer who would also manage our social media platforms. Our services were all up and running by the Spring of 2021. One of my dear gym friends was excited to join me and was perfect for my practice. She was a licensed registered dietician, plant-centered, and a nationally certified Pilates instructor. We posted on Facebook and Instagram every week for a year with little feedback. In the summer of 2021, I started the first Walk with a Doc in the Florida Panhandle, and over the next 18 months, only friends joined me, despite posting on multiple local Facebook group pages. I finally discontinued it due to a lack of participation. My dear friend had family issues arise that caused her to step away from our work.

As 2021 ended, it was time to face and conquer my greatest fear—public speaking. For me, the idea of speaking in front of a group caused paralyzing anxiety. However, the critical mission of educating the public about WFPB eating and evidence-based nutrition science drove me to hire a public speaking coach. Learning how to be comfortable talking to crowds was the only way to gain community presence and trust. The work of LM and changing public health was far more important than my fear.

In the summer of 2022, I enrolled in Dr. Rashmi Schramm's coaching course, "The Power Within." We practiced meditation and worked on spiritual development. It was during that time that I became aware of a negative inner voice that caused me to panic before public speaking events. I named this negative voice "Piggy" because she commandeered my spirit and dissipated my positive energy. It was Piggy who interfered with my personal and professional relationships and had me hiding behind the self-descriptives of "shy" and "introverted." It was Piggy who caused me to retreat from people instead of engaging. Piggy was truly my inner demon! Once revealed, she slowly disappeared.

I have been on multiple podcasts and local television shows and have been an invited guest speaker at civic groups and workshops. I regularly seek out opportunities to speak as the message of LM is urgent and clear: The Standard American Diet (SAD) is literally killing us. There are two types of food, foods that harm and foods that heal.

I started the first LM service in the Florida Panhandle at our clinic that serves the uninsured, the Health and Hope Clinic, LLC. We provide 1:1 nutrition analysis and counseling, and we provide cooking classes in the reception area! We were recently awarded a grant that will provide the resources to bring culinary medicine directly to our local underserved population.

The work in LM has blessed me with many new friendships and business relationships, locally and nationally. They are all wonderfully supportive and helpful. I would not have been able to do this without them.

LM radically changed my life. Whole food plant-centered eating improved my health, improved my family's health, helped me lose 45 pounds, and taught me how to cook and cut sugar cravings. It has been the answer to feeling great as I journey through my 60s. I have gratitude for every day and gratitude for finding the key to feeling younger and stronger for the rest of my days!

Lifestyle Medicine IS the answer to help people lose weight naturally, eat a truly healthy diet, discover intuitive eating, and prevent, arrest, and potentially reverse chronic diseases. Lifestyle Medicine opens the door for all to enjoy their best health.

Lifestyle Medicine brings hope and health back to the practice of medicine. The future is bright!

This chapter is dedicated to my parents, my husband Steve, and my family. Their unconditional love has been the greatest blessing in my life. I am grateful for all of my dear friends and patients, who have also shared their love and support so generously through the years. There are no words to describe my gratitude.

RESOURCES

Documentaries:

Forks Over Knives

The Game Changers

Websites:

Forks Over Knives | Plant-Based Living | Official Website. (2023, May 18). Forks Over Knives. https://www.forksoverknives.com/ with free recipes and plant-centered nutrition information

Plant-Based Nutrition. eCornell. https://ecornell.cornell.edu/certifica tes/nutrition/plant-based-nutrition/ offers one of the best Plant-Based Nutrition educational and certificate programs.

RECIPES. Plant Powered Metro New York. https://www.plantpower edmetrony.org/recipes.html has free plant-centered recipes and an app for your phone.

Dr. Esselstyn's Prevent & Reverse Heart Disease Program | Make yourself heart attack proof. https://www.dresselstyn.com/ for his program and recipes for Preventing and Reversing Heart Disease.

Dr. Yami Cazorla-Lancaster. Dr. Yami Cazorla-Lancaster. https://w ww.doctoryami.com/ provides a pediatrician's perspective, her book is great reading for everyone(see below).

Greger, M. *Nutrition Facts.* Nutrition Facts. https://nutritionfacts.org/ provides well-researched scientific nutrition information with resources by Michael Greger, M.D.

Books:

Cazorla-Lancaster, Y. (2019). *A Parent's Guide to Intuitive Eating: How to Raise Kids Who Love to Eat Healthy.* Simon and Schuster.

Ornish, D., MD, & Ornish, A. (2019). *Undo It!: How Simple Lifestyle Changes Can Reverse Most Chronic Diseases*. Ballantine Books.

Bulsiewicz, W., MD. (2022). *The Fiber Fueled Cookbook: Inspiring Plant-Based Recipes to Turbocharge Your Health*. Penguin.

Adams, E. (2020). *Healthy at Last: A Plant-Based Approach to Preventing and Reversing Diabetes and Other Chronic Illnesses*. Hay House, Inc. by the Mayor of New York City.

Barnard, N. (2020). *Your Body In Balance: The New Science of Food, Hormones and Health*. Hachette UK.

Frates, B., Plaven, B., Watts, B., Agarwal, N., Dalal, M., & Tollefsen, K. (2020). *The Teen Lifestyle Medicine Handbook: The Power of Healthy Living*. Healthy Learning.

Spitz, A., MD. (2018). *The Penis Book: A Doctor's Complete Guide to the Penis--From Size to Function and Everything in Between*. Rodale Books. ("There are foods that will either keep your cucumber fresh or pickle it." Page 182.)

Tibbits, D. (2020). *Forgive to Live: How Forgiveness Can Save Your Life*.

Podcasts:

"Veggie Doctor Radio" *Podcast — Dr. Yami Cazorla-Lancaster*. (2023, May 21). Dr. Yami Cazorla-Lancaster. https://www.doctoryami.com/podcast.

Greger, M. *Nutrition Facts Podcast*. Nutrition Facts Podcast.

Apple Podcasts. (2023, May 9). *The Medical Fitness Podcast on Apple Podcasts*. https://podcasts.apple.com/us/podcast/the-medical-fitness-podcast/id1678017531 Mr. Jeff Young, Kinesiologist, CSCS, ACSM-EIM; Medicine- Rehab-

Apple Podcasts. (2011, September 6). *Fitness Institute on Apple Podcasts*.

https://podcasts.apple.com/us/podcast/fitness-institute/id414291148.

Physicians Committee for Responsible Medicine. *Exam Room Podcast.* https://www.pcrm.org/podcast.

About Dr. Erin Mayfield, DO, DipABLM, DipAOBOG

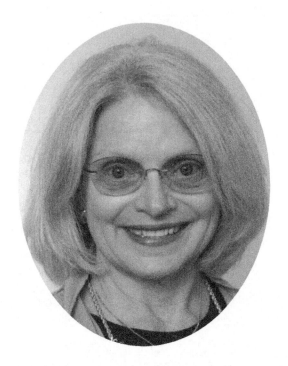

Dr. Erin Mayfield is board certified in Lifestyle Medicine and Obstetrics-Gynecology. She is a Harvard Chef Coach. She is the Founder and CEO of Lifestyle Medicine Wellness and Recovery, LLC, an interactive group coaching practice offering personalized lifestyle interventions and Culinary Medicine classes on a web-based platform. She has over 40 years of experience taking care of patients. Her passion has always been helping people improve their health and resilience using the Six Pillars of Health. Dr. Mayfield started the first Lifestyle Medicine service in the Florida Panhandle, with 1:1 consults and culinary medicine cooking classes. She is a member of numerous professional and civic organizations, including the American College of Lifestyle Medicine and the Teaching Kitchen Collaborative.

Website:

https://LifestyleMedicineWellnessandRecovery.com

Instagram:

https://instagram.com/lifestylemedwellnessrecovery

YouTube:

https://www.youtube.com/@lifestylemedicinewellnessa6351

LinkedIn:

https://www.linkedin.com/in/erin-mayfield-lm-gyn/

Watch an interview with the co-author:

Co-Author spotlight
DR. ERIN MAYFIELD

Scan Me

16

Plant-Based Gut Health Is a Crucial Factor In Controlling Chronic Gastrointestinal Inflammatory Conditions

Khyati Mehta, MD, DipABLM

"Nothing will benefit human health and increase the chances for survival of life on Earth as much as the evolution to a vegetarian diet."

— Albert Einstein

G rowing up in India, the home of Ayurveda, yoga, and vegetarianism, I spent my childhood winter breaks swinging on banyan tree roots in rural India at my grandparents' home. My grandparents lived well into their 90s. When I look back, I know why . . . They ate plants, exercised daily, ate well, and slept well.

I watched my professional parents do the same. I remember practicing yoga with my mom after school and going on long evening walks. In

2002, when I was in medical school, my interest in diverse cultural diets grew. I completed a pediatric residency in India and learned about the basics of nutrition and how to evaluate malnutrition in children. I distinctly remember a seven-month-old baby who was irritable, failing to thrive, and had a large head with frontal bossing. There were concerns about head trauma causing bleeding and hence a large head and discussion about obtaining a head CT scan. His mother was very loving and exclusively breastfeeding. On examining the baby, I immediately knew he had rickets. This is a condition wherein there is a nutritional deficiency of vitamin D, especially in breastfed children. Breast Milk is deficient in vitamin D, and breastfed infants need supplemental vitamin D. My attending physician was very pleased with my diagnosis, and I was so thrilled to be able to help the child with a simple intervention of vitamin D. The child thrived and achieved all milestones thereafter. This and many other cases solidified my passion for nutrition.

Further training in gastroenterology and nutrition seemed to be the obvious next step to harness my love for nutrition and how best to feed the gut. However, this advanced training was not offered at that time in India, and I would have to travel abroad to pursue this fellowship and need to repeat my pediatric residency in the USA, which I did. Ultimately, I spent six years doing two pediatric residencies, one in India and one in America. I was fortunate to learn a good mix of Eastern and Western diets and practices. My topmost priority was to keep learning and educating myself to be a good pediatrician, focusing on nutrition to optimize growth and promote development and well-being.

I completed three additional grueling years of pediatric gastroenterology fellowship. I learned about macronutrients, micronutrients and how best to combine them for a well-balanced diet with adequate carbohydrates, fats, and protein. I also learned about intravenous (IV) nutrition (which was not common in India during my training) and wrote several total parenteral nutrition orders for our sickest patients with inflammatory bowel disease and premature kids who were not ready to eat on their own yet. I absorbed it all and was ready for my journey as a "whole-minded" physician . . . only to be proven wrong a few years into practice. I will elaborate on this below.

As for myself, during this training journey, I had given up on a piece of my own health and well-being as I was working 100-hour work-weeks. I was stress eating a Western diet that was very different from my childhood plant-based diet. As a result, I developed visceral fat that was compounded by my pregnancies, and I had forgotten to exercise as I never had enough time in a day. I knew I had to change for the better, but I kept putting it off until I had more time to change.

After fellowship, I enjoyed my practice and my patients. I continued to make different observations about diet, lifestyle, and exercise and how they played a role in preventing flares or not . . . of the chronic inflammatory gastrointestinal conditions that my patient population had. Eighty percent of my patients felt that good nutrition was essential to their inflammatory bowel disease (IBD) management, and about forty percent believed that diet could control their symptoms. I noticed that my meat-eating patients tended to have longer inflammatory flares of Crohn's disease or ulcerative colitis. However, many of my meat-eating patients ate only a few vegetables or lentils and struggled with foods to eat. I was worried that certain food avoidances in these children could lead to malnutrition. Slowly but steadily, I taught my patients to avoid pro-inflammatory foods—substitute red meat (which is a rich source of protein, iron, vitamin B12, and zinc) with tofu, eggs, bean purees, and lentils. In addition, I advised substituting gluten (a source of fiber, iron, and B vitamins) with rice/oats, substituting dairy (a source of protein, calcium, vitamin D, and potassium) with plant-based milk and fruits like bananas, apples, some citrus foods, and substitute raw cruciferous vegetables like cauliflower, broccoli, and onions for more soft vegetables like squashes and boiled vegetable soups. In people with strictures of their small intestine, a smaller particle size of food is better tolerated than a larger size; for example, applesauce is better tolerated than apples, hummus in place of garbanzo beans, and fruit and vegetable smoothies in place of raw vegetables in salads or berries. I spent hours with my patients going over diet and nutrition in addition to discussing strong immunomodulators and biologic medications for inflammatory bowel disease, as I know well that good nutrition is crucial to gut healing.

I listened to Drs. John Kelly, Caldwell Esselstyn, and Dean Ornish, and I read their books, educating myself about the pillars of Lifestyle Medicine (LM). I learned that most leading authorities like the Food and Agriculture Organization (FAO), World Health Organization (WHO), and World Cancer Research Fund (WCRF) agree that our diets should be primarily plant-based. After about two years of self-education, I decided to take Lifestyle Medicine boards and aced them. This has been the best feather on my cap of accomplishments so far. Traditional medicine taught me to treat chronic diseases, but LM teaches me about healthy lifestyle habits that prevent disease and disease flares. I have indeed come full circle, and I want to impart these good habits to everyone I meet along this journey of life.

I have been able to help myself and thousands of my patients achieve better health with a predominantly plant-based diet. While change is hard and especially so at an early age, I have had some phenomenal results in obese children struggling to eat a healthier, unprocessed diet. A 16-year-old adolescent girl came to me terrified with a diagnosis of non-alcoholic fatty liver disease. She was determined to lose weight and help her liver. She was addicted to soda after every meal and French fries 3–4 times a week. Her lipids, liver enzymes, and insulin levels were high. She was committed to change, and within two weeks of implementing my lifestyle medicine action plan, she started eating better, lost 20 pounds, and was so happy to be running five times a week. Her liver enzymes normalized, and so did her cholesterol and triglycerides.

Another avenue of education is my position as a teaching pediatric gastroenterologist at Loma Linda University in California, which is a large, busy academic center. Loma Linda, CA, is one of the blue zones of the world—a place where people live the longest in the world and where some of the founders of Lifestyle Medicine, like Dr. John Kelly, trained and practiced for years. I incorporate LM practices during my daily rounds. I have taught resident doctors to cook simple, easy recipes so they don't have to put their health off until after training. It brings me immense joy to be the mama bear at work.

So why go plant-based? For several reasons condensed here:

A plant-based diet can reduce the number of medications needed to treat chronic disease including improved digestion, sleep, general health, and sense of well-being. According to an analysis of risk factors from 1990–2010, the leading cause of death and disability in the US was a poor diet which is low in fruits, vegetables, and nuts, and high in processed foods rich in saturated fats. Research has shown that plant-based diets are rich in complex carbohydrates, fiber, and water and lower in energy density. As a result, plant-based diets cause increased satiety and increased resting energy expenditure, which in turn helps with weight loss and healthy weight maintenance. Vegetarians have half the risk of developing diabetes mellitus than non-vegetarians. Some of the benefits to the environment are water conservation, reduced greenhouse gas emissions and carbon footprint of humans, a decrease in waste pollution, and an overall improvement in world hunger.

I will end by saying I am committed to practicing and teaching the pillars of LM. With the recent White House conference on Hunger, Nutrition, and Health goals for our nation and the American College of Lifestyle Medicine's pledge to donate $24.1M to the nutrition training of medical professionals, I am excited for our healthy future. With love and passion, I will continue to help everyone in their journey to better health. Children are little sponges that learn fast and are a joy to teach. I want to reach out to as many children as I can to teach them how to eat well and live an exemplary life. This is what I love to do! Please do not hesitate to contact me with any questions if you want help for your family members or an educational seminar for your community.

This chapter is dedicated to all my patients and their parents for entrusting me with the care of their precious littles. Being a doctor to little kids is hard, but seeing that I can make an impact on children's lives pushes me to learn and grow each day at work.

Many thanks to my loving parents for instilling the love and discipline in me to do great things and to my ever-supportive husband and kids! You are my champions. I love you all.

About Dr. Khyati Mehta, MD, DipABLM

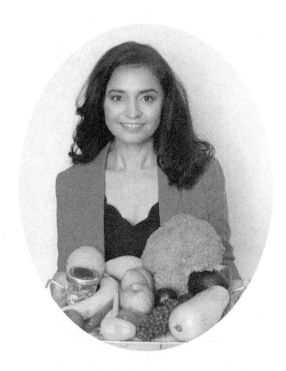

Dr. Khyati Mehta is triple board certified in Pediatrics, Pediatric Gastroenterology, and Lifestyle Medicine. She is faculty at Loma Linda University Medical Center, California, and teaches medical students and residents. With her Eastern roots, she is familiar with the benefits of Ayurveda and yoga for good health. With her Western and LM training, she is enthusiastic and passionate about prevention and staying up to date on treatments needed by her patients with chronic inflammatory gastrointestinal and liver conditions. In addition, she loves traveling and learning new plant-based recipes from diverse cultures all over the globe.

Website: https://lluh.org/provider/mehta-khyati

Instagram: https://instagram.com/thegreengutdoc/

LinkedIn: https://www.linkedin.com/in/khyati-mehta-50023a37/

Watch an interview with the co-author:

DR. KHYATI MEHTA

Scan Me

17

MY PATH TO HEALTH

Anjali Nakra, MBBS, DipIBLM

"A healthy man wants a thousand things, a sick man wants one."

— Confucius

W E had a dream, me, and my father. We both wanted me to become a doctor. And he was so happy when I was admitted to the prestigious Maulana Azad Medical College in Delhi. A year later, one fateful morning, I lost him to serial heart attacks. Diagnosed immediately by his doctor, he walked into an ER, only to collapse soon after arriving there. Why? That question was to become my mission in life. No one should lose their father at the age of 18 years old. This belief became my driving force.

Maybe the cause was his sweet tooth and fondness for fried food . . . . Stress could have been another contributor. Another realization that stuck me was that most of my family is clinically overweight. Maybe, it was the extra weight that contributed to his death. I vowed never to gain weight. Fortunately, this was the easiest part of my journey. As I understood: whatever our genes, keeping a check on weight or relevant parameters is important and manageable. This is what experts say- "Genetics loads the gun, lifestyle pulls the trigger." After my medical degree, I opted for ophthalmology as a specialization but soon realized that was not what I wanted and switched to family practice (FP) immediately, which was closer to my mission.

A few years later, my mother was diagnosed with Type 2 Diabetes. Having lost her younger sibling to diabetes complications, she was cautious and managed her blood glucose well. She was on oral medication for diabetes, despite being careful about her diet and being well-controlled. After an attack of pancreatitis, she decreased her food and oil intake drastically. She lost weight and REVERSED her diabetes, years before Roy Taylor and others proved the link between weight loss and diabetes reversal. I saw my first case of diabetes reversal in my mother. She remained diabetes-free for more than a decade, until her last breath. This was my second lesson, change your lifestyle, and you can achieve reversal or remission of many diseases.

My quest to find all the answers was not easy in the pre-internet era. But I was sure food, stress, and movement were significant. I read journals, took courses, and read a lot of books. With the availability of the internet, it became easier. I read and listened to Dr. T. Colin Campbell, Dr. Michael Gregor, Dr. Dean Ornish, Dr. Herbert Benson, Dr. Neal Bernard, and many more, and finally landed in Boston during the summer of 2013 for a Conference on Lifestyle Medicine (LM). Finally, there was a name for what I wanted to do, and it was evidence-based medicine. Eager to understand the four key factors—nutrition, exercise, sleep, and stress—I attended, soaking up knowledge, and became a member of the American College of Lifestyle Medicine (ACLM). I started to give lifestyle advice to my patients. However, I found It was difficult to give lifestyle advice to patients in their routine Family Practice consultation so, eventually, I started a dedicated LM practice.

In 2018, I attended the Institute of Lifestyle Medicine conference in Boston again, further inspired by Dr. Eddie Philips, Dr. Beth Frates, Dr. Herbert Benson, Dr. Dean Ornish, and Margret Moore—to name a few. I was charged up to come back to India and implement my new knowledge. My family motivated me to take the board certification exam, and I accepted the challenge in the same year. By the end of 2018, I was board certified in Lifestyle Medicine, getting the highest score in my cohort.

Around that time, I developed unexplained fatigue, weight loss, vague abdominal and joint pains, and low-grade fevers. Undergoing multiple scans, blood tests, and even a pet scan was draining. My final diagnosis was panniculitis. I looked for the cause of inflammation in my diet. My food intolerance test revealed intolerance to gluten, dairy, eggs, some nuts, etc., and within weeks of stopping these items, I was back to normal, feeling better and more energetic than ever. It was difficult to give up some of my favorite nuts and dairy, but I managed to make peace with my taste buds, changing them to "health buds" (as my son puts it). Another lesson, our bodies are constantly evolving, and by being perceptive to any changes, we can preempt many conditions.

The Pillars of Lifestyle Medicine

Food as medicine, or lack of nutritious food as disease?

Food is essential for all of us, but abundance and packaged food have changed the way we eat. What, how, and how much we eat gives us oxidative stress, inflammation, and promotes insulin resistance. The wrong food also changes our gut microbes, which aggravates these processes of inflammation. Unfortunately, our relationship with food has changed. We eat when we are celebrating, and we eat when we are sad. Fad diets are even worse. It is crucial to change our relationship with food and to be mindful of what we are putting in our mouths and how our bodies will process the food. A fruit or a vegetable will give us nourishment, bringing down our inflammatory load, versus a serving of fries that will increase inflammation and inflammatory markers (CRP) in minutes.

Traditional Indian diets are carbohydrate (grain) and fat intense. If we manage portions of these two groups, we have an ideal plate. Dairy is also an important part of the meal in India. Most Indian snacks are deep-fried. These two categories (dairy and fried food) are difficult to change for many people.

Further, globalization has led to the introduction of many cuisines and tickled our palates. While it is a positive step, India has more than its share of pasta, pizza, and hamburgers. The occasional chips fried at home have been replaced with a pack a day for most children. Aerated or carbonated drinks, which were occasional, have become more popular than ever. Diet versions of aerated drinks ameliorate the guilt of having excess calories for people, however, those have their own problems. Dietary struggle is real for adults and children alike. Pizza has become the preferred food as compared to chapati/rice with vegetables and dal, by a sizable percentage of the population.

Eating sensibly is the important thing. Eat more whole foods, fruits and vegetables, beans, nuts, and seeds. Avoid inflammatory foods, calorie-dense foods, and packaged foods. It is important to focus on how one feels after a particular food/meal and understand the cues to your best health. My personal experiences and learning from patients have convinced me that there is no one-size-fits-all when it comes to food. Whether it is one of my patients telling me that "I put on weight when I take tomatoes, sorghum, or oats," it all makes sense. After all, this is the era of Precision Medicine, or as Roy C. Ziegelstein puts it—"Personomics."

Exercise as Medicine

Like food, there has been an unfortunate change in the way we move. Regular physical activity has decreased at the population level for all age groups. In the ICMR-INDIAB-5 study, of the individuals studied, 54.4% were inactive, 31.9% were active and 13.7% were highly active. Also, more than 90% of the individuals studied did not participate in any recreational physical activity. Physical movement is much more impactful on our bodies than just calories spent; it is about gaining life, being smarter, and preventing diseases.

Exercise can be addictive, but so can sedentary behavior. To help people start moving, we need to impact more than people's personal choices, we need to change their environment and culture as well. Exercise is important at any and every age, but the two extreme age groups are most vulnerable to the lack of exercise. The majority of children do not get enough opportunities or encouragement to exercise. On the other extreme, the elderly need to exercise to maintain their muscle mass and strength. However, exercise education and awareness are lacking for a majority of them as well.

Sleep as Medicine

Sleep is important for physical, mental, and psychological health. Not only do our bodies need the right number of hours, but also the routine of bedtimes. Delayed sleep and "social jetlag" have a great impact on the molecular reactions of our cells, compounding the lack of an ideal sleep duration of 7–8 hours for adults. *Sleep should be emphasized as a vital sign!* Creating awareness about the impact of a good night's sleep, especially for children and teenagers, will have long-term benefits on their health and growth. Sleep education will affect this age group significantly as they often struggle with adequate sleep duration and nighttime routines.

Stress Management as Medicine

People use the word "Stress" often in day-to-day conversations, not re-alizing the havoc it plays on our bodies physically, mentally, and emotionally. Stress reactions instantly change the way our body functions. The "fight-or-flight" response, which was protective for humans and was followed by "Rest and Digest" recovery, has often become a con-tinuous process now. This chronic stress puts people at risk for obesity, diabetes, heart disease, high blood pressure, dementia, and even some cancers. "Relaxing" or focusing or mindfulness, whatever name we give this process, increases our resilience, suggesting *stress management is as important as the air we breathe or the food we eat*. It is a vital pillar of LM. Managing stress helps us work on eating, exercising, and sleeping better. The term "mind-body medicine" sums it up well, emphasizing that stress impacts our brain and bodies equally.

In their paper, Davies et al defined The lifestyle balance model as: ". . . the degree of equilibrium that exists in one's daily life between the variety of activities a person engages in and the effects of those activities on one's level of health and well-being (. . .) lifestyle balance refers to the amount of stress in a person's daily life compared with stress-reducing activities [and] . . . is also related to diet, social relationships, and spiritual endeavors." This is the power of managing stress.

Managing Substance Use Disorders

Addictions also often begin during stressful periods. Smoking and alcohol use disorders are behaviors, which are the most common forms of addiction. Substance/drug abuse is also commonly seen. In the last few decades, food addiction and excessive screen time have also become all too common. Addictions often coexist with mental health issues. Along with mental health specialists, lifestyle modifications are the foundation of managing all of them. Lifestyle modifications can be as powerful as medications in mild to moderate depression and anxiety disorders.

Social Connections for Health

Social connectedness has emerged as the most important factor for longevity. Social connections are also a great buffer for managing stressful situations. Higher oxytocin levels and lower cortisol levels are found in people who have strong social support systems. Additionally, social connectedness has a positive impact on immune responses. Lack of social connections increases stress levels and adversely impacts heart health and other chronic diseases. The Grant Study of Adult Development at Harvard has established the relationship between social connections, happiness, and longevity beyond doubt.

Patient Transformations

There are many patient stories of the transformative power of lifestyle medicine. I'm sharing two of them that highlight the commitment to changing their lifestyle resulting in success and making our journey a memorable one.

Mrs. N came to lose weight and was ready to change her lifestyle. Her lipids, CRP, and fasting insulin were high, and her life had high-stress levels too.

She was addicted to diet sodas and needed one after each meal. She agreed on decreasing these to half, and within 4–6 weeks, she was able to stop them completely except for an odd day. Potatoes were another favorite. For exercise, she preferred to walk. Within a few weeks of implementing a LM action plan, she would walk at a moderate pace for an hour many times a week. She went to bed late on a regular basis and, for personal reasons, could not change it to optimal levels. Managing stress was a work in progress. By setting goals and working on behavior change, she lost 26 kg in nine months—losing the last few kilograms without any guidance. She had changed her lifestyle!!

Mr. K approached me, "Doc, can I avoid medications for diabetes?" He had already struggled for six months and could bring down his HbA1c a little. I shared LM research in layman's language. Although a self-proclaimed foodie, he was ready to try. We worked together, finding alternatives to deep-fried and oily dishes. The prescription for increasing activity was easy for him as he loved to walk and play sports. Another behavior change that worked was managing portions, especially when eating unhealthy dishes. Sleep and stress were also managed well by setting goals. Sleep scheduling and achieving seven hours of sleep were easily managed by him. Three months later, his HbA1c had improved to prediabetes levels. Making changes is easier with a clear goal in mind.

What I Have Learned from My Patients

Patients who have changed their lifestyles for good and those who have not been able to achieve their targets have taught me a lot. Curriculum and courses are the foundation of our skills as LM physicians, but what I have learned from patients has added immensely to my skills. Focusing not only on the "what" but the "why" should I change is equally important. Once we help patients identify their why, it is easier to work on the how. Making minor changes can go a long way in changing overall health, especially if they come from patients themselves. Behavior change techniques are a vital part of a lifestyle consultation, walking with them, and guiding them helps to make change easier for patients, and gratifying for me.

Lifestyle Medicine is the new paradigm in healthcare. Health and wellness are the focus. The new approach of treating a person as a whole, focusing on improving health, physical, mental, and emotional, has far more impact than treating a disease. It's transforming a person! With lifestyle-related noncommunicable diseases being 70% of the disease burden of our world, we need to work on the root cause of chronic disease, which is lifestyle. I am grateful to be a part of this change in healthcare for my family and my patients, and the world.

This chapter is dedicated to my parents, whose unconditional love was and is my strength, and to my family, who have encouraged me to follow my passion.

References:

Davies, G., Elison, S., Ward, J. M., & Laudet, A. B. (2015). The role of lifestyle in perpetuating substance use disorder: the Lifestyle Balance Model. *Substance Abuse Treatment Prevention and Policy, 10*(1). https ://doi.org/10.1186/1747-597x-10-2.

Ziegelstein, R. C. (2015). Personomics. *JAMA Internal Medicine, 175*(6), 888. https://doi.org/10.1001/jamainternmed.2015.0861.

Anjana, R. M., Das, A., Deepa, M., Bhansali, A., Joshi, S. R., Joshi, P., Dhandhania, V. K., Rao, P. V., Sudha, V., Subashini, R., Unnikrishnan, R., Madhu, S. V., Kaur, T., Mohan, V., & Shukla, D. (2014). Physical activity and inactivity patterns in India – results from the ICMR-IN-DIAB study (Phase-1) [ICMR-INDIAB-5]. International Journal of Behavioral Nutrition and Physical Activity, 11(1). https://doi.org/10. 1186/1479-5868-11-26.

Vaillant, George E.; McArthur, Charles C.; Bock, Arlie, 2022, "Grant Study of Adult Development, 1938-2000", https://doi.or g/10.7910/DVN/48WRX9, Harvard Dataverse, V4, UNF:6:FfCN-PD1m9jk950Aomsriyg== [fileUNF].

Begum, S., Hinton, E. C., Toumpakari, Z., Frayling, T. M., Howe, L., Johnson, L., & Lawrence, N. (2023). Mediation and moderation of genetic risk of obesity through eating behaviours in two UK cohorts. International Journal of Epidemiology. https://doi.org/10.1093/ije/d yad092

About Dr. Anjali Nakra, MBBS, DipIBLM

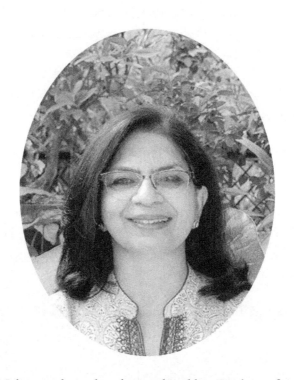

Dr. Anjali Nakra graduated and completed her Diploma from Maulana Azad Medical College and associated LNJPN Hospital, GB Pant Hospital, and Guru Nanak Eye Centre, New Delhi. She worked with the Ministry of Health, Abu Dhabi, UAE, following which she started a Family Practice in Delhi. She has completed various certifications in Evidence-Based Diabetes Management, Clinical Research Methods, Fundamentals of Mind-Body Medicine, Motivational interviewing, etc. She is certified in Obesity Management by the World Obesity Federation. She has a special interest in obesity and behavior change. She is a member of the Indian Medical Association, Delhi Medical Association, ACLM, Indian Society of Lifestyle Medicine (ISLM), and RSSDI and has been the past Secretary and Executive Committee Member of ISLM.

Instagram: https://www.instagram.com/pathtohealthclinic/

Facebook: https://www.facebook.com/dranjalinakra/

LinkedIn: https://www.linkedin.com/in/anjali-nakra-9a6a87b5/

Website: www.pathtohealthclinic.com

Watch an interview with the co-author:

Co-Author spotlight
DR. ANJALI NAKRA

Scan Me

18

PHYSICIAN, HEAL THYSELF

Lisa Pathak, MD, FACP, FAAP, DipABLM

"We are born in one day. We die in one day. We can change in one day. And we can fall in love in one day. Anything can happen in just one day."

— Gayle Forman

I believe that those of us who go into the medical field truly do so to help **other** people, cure disease, and relieve suffering. Those who go into the field of Lifestyle Medicine do so for different reasons. I don't know a single physician who is practicing in this field who wasn't drawn into it, first and foremost, to heal **themselves.** I am no exception.

The year was 2020. I was 47 years old, raising my three daughters, managing my busy primary care private practice, and doing all the hard things—dealing with a stressful marriage, serving in the Air Force reserves, working on creating our "nest egg" to ensure a happy retirement, saving for college tuition, and assisting in our real estate investing. To say I was a bit overwhelmed is an understatement! In order to deal with this amount of cognitive stress, I tapped into my ancestral roots a few years earlier and started a daily meditative practice. Although I didn't know anyone personally practicing meditation, I had grown up hearing all about the power of meditation and how Yogis can control their own blood pressure and brain waves with breathwork.

I decided to start with 10 minutes in the morning of guided meditation with breathwork and noticed my "monkey mind" started to calm. I quickly progressed to 10 minutes twice a day, as I saw tangible results. Meditation helped me to learn how to manage my thoughts and my mind. It helped me to become less reactive, more intentional, and present in the moment. I also started noticing the simple things I had taken for granted, like the colorful sunrises and the radiant smiles of my daughters. After a few months of dedicated practice, I also found myself welcoming and looking for gratitude in my daily life.

As the pandemic hit in March 2020 and office hours decreased, I suddenly had some extra time on my hands. This resulted in some extra bandwidth to start exploring. It was then that I discovered the field of Lifestyle Medicine (LM) from a social media group. Until this point, I had never heard of Lifestyle Medicine, despite being a board-certified internist and pediatrician.

I was immediately intrigued! Although meditation was life-changing for me, I felt I needed more. I wasn't exactly sure what "more" was at the time. But as I was approaching my late 40s, the aging process was really starting to hit home. By this point in my career, I had witnessed thousands of seniors age with loss of function, disability, pain, and loneliness. I was determined that I definitely did not want to go out like that. I was interested in healthy aging and optimal living. I wasn't looking for the newest supplement, procedure, or gadget but true optimal living from the inside out.

Surprisingly, this was the first time in my life that I was consciously choosing my own health as a priority. My personal health had always been the last thing on my mind. I reflected on how a physician could make his or her own personal health an afterthought and realized that it's probably a similar story for most high-performing, driven professionals.

As a young adult, my dream was to become a physician; I dedicated countless hours and days of sitting and studying, not to mention the occasional semi-all-nighters during exam weeks. This rigorous schedule involved caffeine, sugar, and junk food, keeping me up at night and allowing me the bragging rights that I could study that long.

It didn't get easier after graduating from medical school, however. Residency meant 36-hour shifts every 3–4 nights, combined with presentations, studying, and clinical work. There was no time or energy left for exercise, social interactions, or nutritious meals. I was on autopilot, trying to get to the next point. However, I soon realized the next point didn't get better either.

After residency, I was still working 80-hour weeks in my first job. I quickly realized my schedule wasn't sustainable and changed jobs. But soon thereafter, I started having my children—three girls, all roughly two years apart. I continued working and mothering. After getting frustrated with the administration at the local hospital, I decided to take the plunge and open my own practice. With that decision came a great deal of additional responsibility and stress. After a few years of growing the practice to profitability, my husband and I realized that we needed tax-sheltering investments going further, which started our real estate investing journey. So as you can see, it never ends—my own personal health and self-care were never on the agenda, nor was it for my husband, for that matter.

I began to see many of my own friends and colleagues of similar ages battling autoimmune disease, arthritic pain, heart disease, and even cancer. I often wondered how I was able to escape it, despite not making my health a priority and experiencing a tremendous amount of daily stress and responsibility. In hindsight, I definitely attribute my overall health to three things.

First and foremost, I consider myself lucky to be born into an Indian family that practiced much of the ancestral wisdom passed down through the generations. This included following a vegetarian diet. Although I grew up avoiding many of the traditional inflammatory foods, my diet wasn't ideal either. I didn't necessarily eat the most nutritious foods, as many of our meals were processed, carbohydrate-based, and fried in oil.

The second thing that I feel helped me to avoid chronic illnesses early on was being in the US Air Force Reserves with its arduous physical fitness requirements. Every year a PT test is required, which involves a timed run, push-ups, and sit-ups. This requirement basically forced us to stay active and exercise, and it also became a community builder. A few of us would pass fitness tips back and forth in addition to working out after drills together. Although I hated the run, the fear of the PT test made me exercise.

The third thing that kept me healthy was my daily meditation practice, which I had been doing consistently since my early 40s. My meditative practice had expanded over the years, starting out with guided meditations and breathwork and expanding to different Buddhist meditations and Vedic mantra-based meditations. As of today, I continue to practice and explore different modalities of mindfulness and meditation.

So, I had been practicing some aspects of at least three of the pillars of Lifestyle Medicine all along, without even realizing it! I continued to absorb all the content from the Lifestyle Medicine course, fully aware that I needed to do more. I had been holding an extra 15 pounds of post-pregnancy weight for many years, and I could definitely see the effects of aging on my face and hair. I was ready to make myself a priority.

I loved learning new information and enjoyed the new friendships I was making with like-minded people. My only regret was I wish I had learned these things 20 years earlier! One of the factors which really helped me be more accountable was joining a LM-inspired accountability group called "Mindfully Healthy" with friends and colleagues. We would track our individual goals and share wins and frustrations. It was amazing to have that kind of support from friends and colleagues with similar lifestyle-related goals.

I was most surprised by the evidence that the quality of your social connections determines longevity, as it was proven by the famous Harvard study from 1938. It really opened my eyes to how my relationships had also taken a back burner. I always planned to call or get together with loved ones after completing certain tasks, almost like a reward. However, since the tasks didn't get completed, I would never get around to calling. *All along, I thought of "catch-up" time as a luxury, not a necessity.* After learning the evidence about the importance of social connections, I prioritize my most important relationships as a necessity for my health and devote the required effort to it with eagerness. The results have been far-reaching as they contagiously inspired others to do the same.

Although I had tremendous personal results following the pillars of Lifestyle Medicine, I questioned whether my patients would be open to change. I practice in a rural "meat and potatoes" type of area. I didn't know if my patients were truly ready or interested in making lifestyle changes. "Physician, heal thyself" is a proverb that describes the mentality that "we won't believe what you are saying unless you can prove that it works using yourself as the example."

After becoming board certified in Lifestyle Medicine, I decided to put it to the test. I started by asking my patients for more detailed information on nutrition, physical activity, water intake, sleep, and the status of their social connections and loneliness. I began offering them one or two action items that they could work on with each visit. To my surprise, this exchange was exactly what patients were looking for! They all wanted to know what they could or should be doing. They wanted to get off medications or at least decrease some of them. Most importantly, they wanted to feel vibrant and healthy again. I was shocked by the results I was getting! Day after day, patient after patient, I was amazed and encouraged by the transformations I was seeing.

For example, a patient with chronic kidney disease that I had been following for years stopped eating meat, increased his fruits, vegetables, and water intake, and started exercising again. He came back three months later with normal kidney function—without any other therapeutic intervention!

Another significant case that stands out is a 60-year-old female's follow-up after she was hospitalized due to a suicide attempt. After one interaction with me, she left fully transformed. Whereas with this type of visit, I would have normally discussed talk therapy, medication, side effects, and possibly a psychiatry referral, I decided to use a Lifestyle Medicine approach to the appointment. After 40 minutes of asking Lifestyle Medicine-related questions and using some motivational interviewing techniques, she decided to start making green smoothies in the morning and return to water aerobics and crocheting . . . activities which brought her joy. She also decided to call her friends from church who she used to lunch with pre-COVID and convince them to restart their get-togethers. She left the office smiling and invigorated, with a new zest for life. I couldn't believe the impact! I don't ever remember making such a profound impact on a depressed patient in such a short time in my entire career. At that point, I knew I was onto something, and this was going to be my path.

My individual appointments soon scaled to shared medical appointments, where I would see 10–12 patients at a time, teaching them valuable lifestyle medicine skills and inspiring them to make tangible changes. This transpired because I couldn't keep up with the demands and didn't feel right about withholding such life-changing education from deserving patients. It made the most sense to share this information in a group setting. The results were nothing short of miraculous. After six weeks, we had individual patients with sensational results, including 22-pound weight loss, 2 inches slimmer abdominal circumference, significantly improved depression and anxiety as demonstrated on baseline scoring evaluations, HgA1c improved by 2 points, and one particular patient was able to decrease his triglycerides by 600 points by implementing these changes without any medication changes.

I was so excited with the results I was getting that I decided to share the information with my medical group in the Air Force Reserves. I gave a presentation on Lifestyle Medicine and introduced the concept of "blue zones." Blue zones are areas of the world where people live the longest lives, consistently reaching age 100. To my surprise, after the presentation, I was swarmed with people coming to my office wanting more information and thanking me for the presentation. I learned from several members that they had been struggling with their own health concerns and not getting answers or results. They all desperately wanted to take control of their own health.

As a result of that single lecture, at least two members of the medical group have completely transformed their lives by changing to a whole food plant-based diet and incorporating all the other lifestyle medicine pillars, resulting in weight loss, getting off medications, reduced pain, and more vitality. I also discovered that Lifestyle Medicine clinics, disguised as "High Performance Clinics," did exist in the Air Force, and there was already an established Lifestyle and Performance Medicine Working Group, which I joined immediately.

I believe I've made a more significant and meaningful impact in the last three years practicing Lifestyle Medicine than in the 20 years prior, and it all started with healing myself first! In transforming my own health, I have been able to motivate and educate my patients, my family, and my friends in their own journey to more healthy, vibrant, and rewarding lives. And I have so much more to give!

———◆○◆———

This chapter is dedicated to my loving parents, who set the foundation for not only most of the pillars of a healthy lifestyle but also nurtured the values of education, self-confidence, grit, integrity, and spirituality.

For this, I am forever grateful and hope to pass their legacy and all the new knowledge I have acquired to my own precious three daughters.

———◆○◆———

About Dr. Lisa Pathak, MD, FACP, FAAP, DipABLM

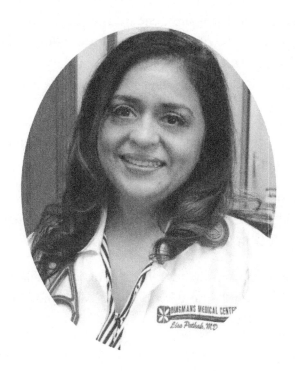

Dr. Lisa Pathak is board certified in Internal Medicine, Pediatrics, and Lifestyle Medicine. She is a graduate of the accelerated seven-year medical program at the Sophie Davis School of Biomedical Education at City College and received her Doctorate of Medicine from Mt. Sinai Medical School in New York City.

She completed her residency at Cooper Hospital/UMDNJ Camden, where she was selected as the Chief Resident during her final year.

Dr. Pathak has earned her Fellowship in both Internal Medicine and Pediatrics. Fellowship is an honorary designation given to recognize ongoing individual service and contribution to the practice of medicine, and thereby a mark of distinction. By maintaining her Fellowship, she makes special efforts to be a better doctor and deliver high-quality healthcare.

She considers herself a lifelong learner with a strong belief in overall wellness and disease prevention, and therefore has expanded her education and became board certified in Lifestyle Medicine in 2020, which is her true calling. Lifestyle Medicine is the study of how our lifestyle choices can prevent, reverse, and treat chronic medical conditions incorporating specific recommendations with nutrition, mental health, physical activity, social connectedness, sleep, and avoidance of harmful substances.

She is the founder of Dingmans Medical, a primary care practice in North East PA, where she incorporates Lifestyle Medicine for all ages, from pediatrics to geriatrics.

In addition to her practice, Dr. Pathak is currently a Lieutenant Colonel in the United States Air National Guard and serves at Stewart Air National Guard Base in Newburgh, NY.

Dr. Pathak is an active member of the American College of Lifestyle Medicine, USAF Lifestyle and Performance Medicine Working Group, and Poplar Care Network.

Dr. Pathak lives in North East Pennsylvania with her family and, in her free time, enjoys hiking, spending time in nature, reading, yoga, traveling, and inspiring conversations. She continues to maintain a daily meditation practice and incorporates an uncluttered minimalist-inspired lifestyle.

Website: https://dingmansmedical.com/

LinkedIn: https://www.linkedin.com/in/lisa-pathak/

<u>Watch an interview with the co-author:</u>

DR. LISA PATHAK

Scan Me

19

Learning How to Live Well: A Physician-Mother-Coach Journey Comes Full Circle

Amy Patel, MD, FAAP, DipABIM, DipABLM

"Living well is an art that can be developed: a love of life and ability to take great pleasure from small offerings and assurance that the world owes you nothing and that every gift is exactly that, a gift."
— Maya Angelou, Wouldn't Take Nothing for My Journey Now

I knew I wanted to be a physician since I was 15 years old. I loved everything about science, and I was an aspirational teenager who wanted to save the world. There was no doubt in my mind that the most important way I could contribute in life was to be a physician, to help people, and to ensure that everyone had access to high quality healthcare.

In my adolescent brain, this profession looked very much like a Normal Rockwell painting, "Doctor and the Doll." I saw this in a wall calendar that my parents had given me, a paper page depicting the painting, printed in an issue of the *Saturday Evening Post* from 1929. In this painting, a physician was examining a girl's doll, building trust with his young patient, who he would guide into excellent health habits for the rest of her life. He had a black bag by his side, which I imagined was filled with all of the necessary tools to monitor a patient's health, diagnose, and treat any health condition they might have. I imagined that her parents were off to the side, watching and listening intently to all of the important advice that this doctor would share with them. While this doctor was an older white man, and I did not have any role models outside of my home who looked like me, there was never a doubt in my mind that I would be just as respected, trusted, and effective as this doctor in this painting.

I was especially drawn to helping those who did not have what I had. My parents immigrated from India to the United States to establish a life they believed would bring opportunities for their future children that would be bigger than their own. On this foundation, my parents made sure that my siblings and I had access to nourishing food, good education, and a safe neighborhood to enjoy the outdoors. I visited India for the first time when I was 11 years old, met dozens of members of my extended family, and saw where my parents grew up. For the first time, I saw poverty and homelessness, something I had not yet seen or known of back home. My curiosity led me to understand that these issues existed almost everywhere, and I began to question what else people did not have that I had previously assumed everyone had. Over the next few years of my adolescence, I learned that some people did not have access to healthcare, and even those who did have access might receive disparate care based on various factors. This was the beginning of my understanding of what I now know as health disparities, healthcare disparities, and social determinants of health. In college, my understanding deepened through my participation in classes focused on community health. I decided I should become a pediatrician and work in underserved areas where my help as a physician was needed the most.

I followed the path I had confidently and clearly laid out in my head—completed college, medical school, and residency. I was a National Health Service Corps scholar, receiving a scholarship to pay for medical school, and in return, I would work in an underserved area after completing my residency. I completed a residency in internal medicine and pediatrics, and my first attending physician position was in a community health center in an urban underserved area. While rewarding in many ways, I quickly realized the numerous systemic challenges in the healthcare field. I was burning out fast, and I had just started my career. I questioned how I could have trained for over 20,000 hours to become a double board-certified physician and feel like the work I was doing was not making a difference in my patients' lives. I spent well over my allotted 15 minutes with each patient, addressing their acute and chronic health issues, and when they followed up, many of them would continue to have the same poor control of their issues. Some never filled their prescriptions because they could not afford to do so or could not afford the transportation to go to the specialist I scheduled them to see. While some resources were available, there were many barriers my patients had to overcome in order to access them. The paperwork, wait times for services to be put in place, low healthcare literacy, an unfamiliar healthcare system, financial stress, lack of access to safe outdoor spaces, and the cost burden of nutrient-dense whole foods were just some of the challenges my patients faced.

I saw the same challenges in primary care, urgent care, and hospital medicine. I spent more time than I had to educate and motivate my patients to change their lifestyle after discharge, and many would return because they resumed their prior health habits when they went home. I was staying late at work, completing patient charts before bed and early in the morning, and I was physically and emotionally exhausted. My own health was suffering as I no longer had time to prioritize exercise, sleep, and social connections, and my stress levels were consistently high.

In 2014, I learned about a field of medicine called Lifestyle Medicine (LM). I read about this with enthusiasm and found a conference to attend. During the conference, I learned from leaders in the field who presented extensive research spanning over four decades on lifestyle interventions that could reduce or prevent the majority of chronic diseases. I interacted with colleagues across many healthcare disciplines who had interesting and innovative approaches in practice—teaching patients how to shop for healthy foods on a budget and cook plant-forward meals, walking with patients, and working in healthcare spaces with integrated care teams focusing on prevention. I was reinvigorated and inspired as this was the way I had envisioned medicine should be practiced. I was hopeful again to know that I was not wrong about medicine. I had found my healthcare people, and I was ready to figure out how to take what I learned to my work with patients. I continued to learn about LM, its principles, the research, and elements that I could integrate into patient care. In 2019, I became a board-certified Lifestyle Medicine physician.

During this time, I led a team of health professionals in a secondary school wellness center. Every student had access to nutritious food, daily exercise, and healthcare services. I shared my excitement about LM and opened the opportunity for my team to become lifestyle medicine practitioners. Several team members became LM practitioners, including our nutritionist, a physician assistant, nurse practitioner, and administrative director. During the pandemic, we expanded our wellness programming and used the six pillars of LM as the main principles. We invited students and school faculty and staff to participate in programs that were virtual at first and later in person. I added LM principles to wellness education, programming, and medical visits with students.

On a personal level, finding LM has helped me be a better role model to my patients and my children. It has served as an anchor when my own health habits became secondary again, like during the pandemic. The plant-based foods from my childhood are what I eat with my family. Exercise and movement are part of daily life. I am able to recognize the profound impact that stress has on my mood and my body. I take time daily to connect with my loved ones. And I give myself the same gentle understanding I give to my patients when my balance is disrupted. Lifestyle Medicine is the foundation that I continue to use for myself.

To complement my work as a LM physician, pediatrician, and internist, I completed a life coach certification in 2022, which has helped me to expand my skill set. The simple way to summarize my approach as a physician-mother-coach is that I help people learn how to live well. Some patients focus on healthy weight management or improving their relationship with substances (and working toward minimizing or avoiding use) or running a marathon. I help patients look at the bigger picture as well and explore what it means to them to live well. One patient told me that she was tired of her weight fluctuating so much—months of eating better and exercising only to drop those habits and gain back the lost weight. I helped her to step back and find her real goal, what was she trying to do by losing weight, and why was the number on the scale her measure of health? After some discussion and thought, she articulated that her goal was to live to see her grandchildren and to be mobile enough to play with her grandchildren when she was older. For her, that is what living well means. Once that was understood, the path to achieving better health was much easier to develop and follow using LM principles as a guide.

My journey to this point has not been as linear or straightforward as I thought it would be when I was a teenager. The healthcare system is more complicated, and systemic barriers make it challenging for patients and the physicians leading their care. While the practice of medicine is not as simple as that Norman Rockwell painting, Lifestyle Medicine has been instrumental in my path to learning how to live well and helping others do the same.

This chapter is dedicated to my parents, who sacrificed so much in life to provide me with the foundation that makes me who I am today, and to my family (Jason, Reese, Maya), who inspire me to be the best version of myself so I can help patients transform their lives through lifestyle medicine and coaching.

About Dr. Amy Patel, MD, FAAP, DipABIM, DipABLM

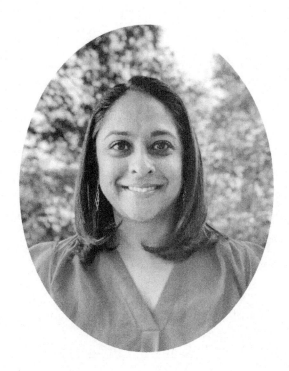

Dr. Amy Patel is a physician and professional coach board certified in Pediatrics, Internal Medicine, and Lifestyle Medicine. She completed her residencies in these programs at the University of Pittsburgh Medical Center and Children's Hospital of Pittsburgh. Dr. Patel earned a BS in Biology and Community Health from Tufts University and her MD degree from the University of Vermont College of Medicine. As a certified coach, she focuses on helping people develop and optimize wellness, leadership, and life skills. Her professional interests are rooted in the belief that everyone deserves access to quality healthcare and evidence-based inclusive health education.

Dr. Patel is also a member of the Sports Medicine Advisory Council for the New England Prep School Athletic Council and a member of the Association of Independent Schools of New England Health and Wellness annual conference planning committee. She has presented at local and national conferences on a variety of topics, such as health and wellness, leadership, and social determinants of health and health disparities. She has conducted school health and health center assessments and helped schools develop their pandemic response plan.

Dr. Patel is currently the Dean of Health and Wellness and Chief Medical Officer at Phillips Academy. She teaches in the Empathy, Balance, and Inclusion course and guest teaches in physical education and biology on health topics, including sexuality and substance use. She also serves as an academic advisor and supports student-led health initiatives as a faculty advisor to several student clubs. She consults across campus on a wide variety of health issues at individual and policy levels. In addition, she is a member of several committees that work to support students and is also an advisor to several student clubs committed to student health and wellness.

In her spare time, Dr. Patel enjoys practicing what she teaches, spending time with family and friends, and traveling throughout the world.

LinkedIn: https://www.linkedin.com/in/amy-patel-54519712?trk=contact-info

Instagram: https://instagram.com/livewellmdcoach/

Watch an interview with the co-author:

Co-Author spotlight
DR. AMY PATEL

Scan Me

20

LIFESTYLE IS MEDICINE

Karmi Patel, MD, FACP, DipABLM

"The doctor of the future will give no medicine, but will interest his patient in the care of the human frame, in diet and in the cause and prevention of disease."

— Thomas Edison

The 'field of medicine' is an appropriate phrase, much more significant than is appreciated in everyday life. Medicine as a profession is vast in its domain and fruitful in practice. Through rigorous reading and research, we, as physicians, plow through the soil that is the world's available raw data, extracting and then replanting it, cultivating our thoughts and ideas. With some time, tender, and continual, progressive attention, the ideas grow and develop, and everyone can enjoy the fruits of our labors.

For myself, 'farming' the 'field' began what seems now a long time ago. Growing up in India, my desire to pursue medicine was inherently strong, pulled by the comfort of aiding people in their sick or painful times. I witnessed the practice of Western medicine married with ancient Ayurvedic remedies for common and chronic conditions. Immigrating to the USA at the age of 16 and earning a Science Award during my undergraduate studies at Penn State University served not only to offer encouragement and motivation but also as a confirmation of my intellectual competence. Youthful idealism gave way to reality as I worked directly with patients and physicians as an Easton Hospital ER intern. I learned the basics of CPR, tying and removing sutures, and listening to heart sounds. This fundamental experience introduced me to an array of emotions which made me realize that the field of medicine embodied more than pure scientific skills, that ultimately, human empathy is the "heart of medicine."

I relished responsibility and challenge and thus decided to continue to grow and develop by seeking the opportunity to put these beliefs into practice in the context of the professional medical environment. I joined Ross University School of Medicine.

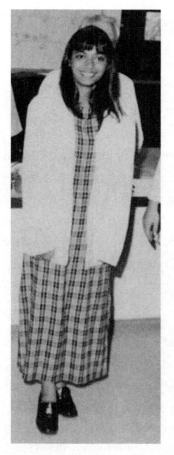

Photo of my white coat ceremony (WCC), September 2000. Donning our new coats, we took our first steps in becoming a 'doctor' by taking the Hippocratic oath, "Primum non nocere (first do no harm)." These words were etched clearly in my memory.

We milled through rich, dense tracts of information, learning about anatomy, physiology, biochemistry, pharmacology, pathology, and ethics. Much of the focus of our education was placed on diagnosing and treating many common conditions. Nutrition and preventing disease were a minimal focus. As a matter of fact, my medical school had only one credit course on nutrition (this deficiency will play an essential part later on). As a student, I studied hard, striving to ensure that I absorbed and understood all the theories and concepts of medical literature, securing my technical proficiency in future practice. Following graduation, I commenced intense years of residency, where we started to implement the knowledge learned under the guidance of our mentors and fellow senior colleagues. After completing an extra year as a chief resident, I decided to join the academic practice at my residency training center.

One day during my routine practice, I saw a 40-year-old male who was referred to me by his work for evaluation of high blood pressure. He had all the risk factors: smoking, being overweight, poor dietary habits, and alcohol use. He had two blood pressure readings that, as defined by the Joint National Criteria, put him at stage 1 hypertension. So, as recommended by guidelines, I took my prescription pad out and wrote for him to take a very commonly used medication:

Hydrochlorothiazide 25 mg

Sig: To take 1 tab daily by mouth

Disp: 30 Refills: 3

The patient was advised of needing to take meds daily, in the mornings, as it may cause increased urination. Additional recommendations included: exercise, close control of his salt intake, and restricting it to 2 grams/day. We discussed the need to do blood work to check his cholesterol, kidney, and liver function. When the results came back, he had high cholesterol, and his fasting sugar was slightly elevated. Because he was recently diagnosed hypertensive with risk factors for cardiovascular disease, he needed to be on cholesterol-lowering medication. Out came the prescription pad again:

Atorvastatin 10 mg

Sig: To take 1 tab at bedtime

Disp: 30 Refills: 3

My additional recommendations extended to following a heart-healthy diet and return for a follow-up visit in three months with labs. Three months later, he had fasting labs which showed his blood sugars were high, and his HbA1c was within diabetic range! All of a sudden, it just hit me! Three months ago, this gentleman was absent from diagnoses; now, I have labeled him with three and started him on three medications. Unfortunately, two of the medications, blood pressure and cholesterol medication, likely caused him to have his third problem! But, wait, I had taken the oath to 'do no harm,' and here I am doing precisely that—unintentionally.

At the same time, in my personal life, we had just welcomed our beautiful baby boy, who had a stomach viral illness at 12 months old. Our pediatrician suggested Gatorade as my baby could not keep Pedialyte down. Since he loved the color red, I picked up red Gatorade, and after drinking that, he developed a rash all over his body! As a mother, I felt guilty of neglect. Here I am, trying to help my baby and instead causing more harm again! Desperate for redemption, my standard of care demanded deep examination and prompted heightened scrutiny of each possible health-related decision.

Wanting to understand the broad components of well-health and its finer details, I looked more into what was in that bottle of Gatorade. What is it that we put in our foods? What are we putting in our bodies? These events began a self-journey of learning more about foods and nutrition. On this path, I realized that in medical school, we were taught about nutrition less than we were about diagnosing and treating diseases with meds. It was not about the prevention of root causes of diseases like diabetes, high blood pressure, and high cholesterol, which are likely lifestyle diseases. So I started cutting out processed foods from our diet and eating more of a Mediterranean diet. I watched many documentaries like "Supersize Me" and "Blue Zones," and one day, I stumbled upon "Forks Over Knives." Hearing Dr. Greger and many other doctors talk about lifestyle and preventing chronic diseases was music to my ears. Simultaneously, one of my interventional cardiology friends had met Dr. Joel Fuhrman and insisted on joining him at the Lifestyle Medicine conference in Arizona.

Attending the American College of Lifestyle Medicine conference both renewed my passion and helped me discover my tribe. It all made sense. I learned about the six pillars at the core of living a long healthy life: whole food plant-based diet, exercise, sleep, stress management, social connectedness, and avoiding risky substances. Naturally, this led to me sitting down for a US-based Lifestyle Medicine certification exam in 2018 and successfully becoming a Diplomate of the American Board of Lifestyle Medicine. Implementing changes in our diet by cutting out dairy and other animal products meant that I no longer had to rely on allergy medication and didn't have my twice-a-year sinus infections. My husband could come off allergy meds and didn't require taking his asthma inhalers. Not to mention, we both lost 20+ lbs and normalized our BMI. It was challenging. We were confronted and mocked by many for being too strict about what we eat. "Everything in moderation." "Little here and there is not going to kill you." "You shouldn't be that hard on kids." However, those taunts stopped as time went by, and they saw us being our healthy selves. My son, unsolicited, became vegan at age 10 for his love of animals. My motivation to continue with a plant-based healthy lifestyle is how energetic my body feels now.

In my past experiences, to get paid, part of my salary was based on the volume of patients seen, tests ordered, referrals made, etc. This model led to hamster-wheel care of routine three-month follow-ups with blood work. However, upon following my advice and making lifestyle changes, many of my patients no longer needed to be seen every three months or get unrequired lab work as their chronic conditions were stable. It was then that I came across reading about the Whole Healthcare approach, which emphasizes care centered around what matters to the patient's well-being. Professionally, I joined Veterans Affairs in Knoxville after my certification upon learning of the VA's implementation of "Whole Health," a program that followed many of the core principles of lifestyle medicine. This transition was the best decision of my career as I can guide Veterans to positive health outcomes, come off medications, and possibly, truly prevent chronic conditions without the burden of billing and generating revenue. Now, I am equipped with a list of foods and lifestyle changes rather than just taking out my prescription pad. I am able to meet where my patients are and help them adjust and adapt to changes that can lead them to healthier lifestyles. I want to share a heartfelt letter that nicely summarized these efforts and the transition to a healthy lifestyle that was written by one of my patients.

①

Dear Dr. Patel,

First of all please forgive me for the printing of this letter, I struggle with a keyboard so my typing abilities suffer. I also want you to feel free to share this letter with anyone you feel can benefit from it and I also don't care if you share my medical records because what is happening and has happen is truly amazing, life changing and it needs to be shared.

I want to start off by saying, my pass exposure to the medical profession was and is how most patients are exposed, "You have this condition we will treat it with this drug." There was not much healing and to be honest, I didn't believe, that most of what I was diagnosed with could ever be reversed. I was told it could be controlled with medication and diet, but never once was I told it could be reversed. This went on for years, pills, pills and more pills. That all changed when you became my physician. You explained that "hey, you can get off these chemicals by just changing your diet." Now I am an old vet, set in my ways, very stubborn, but inside me, I really wanted to be rid of all these medications. I was tired of keeping up with pills, tired of costing tax payers money, tired of being held down taking medication

Letter to Dr. Patel from her patient - Page 1

③

AND waiting for my turn to leave this earth.
So when you explained just give up meat for
awhile and see. Well I thought, what is it going
to hurt to try, I believe I can do it. Well
nobody else thought I could, but you did. I
have spent most of my life, after the Army,
weighing over 300 pounds, excessive drinking, smoking,
I was sprinting toward the grave. My wife, my
friends were like you can't do this, you eat meat
for every meal. But someone believed in me, someone
who was very intelligent, who spent years studying
medicine, the human body, it was my doctor,
doctor Patel. So I did it, first step no meat
for breakfast, then lunch, then dinner. Wow,
I went all day, days turned to weeks, weeks
turned to months. But what really I was feeling
the change was how I began to feel, the way
I began to look. This is working, profoundly!!
I then took futher steps, from just the small talks we
have at my appointments, to practice my breathing.
Major changes were happening, stress is becoming a
thing of the past. You have changed my mindset
from being fixed to a growth mindset. I am
living proof of neoroplasticity, Dr Patel you
have rewired my brain. No longer am I exsisting,
I am living growing, changing into a healthy

Letter to Dr. Patel from her patient - Page 2

③

more productive human being. You are healing
not just treating. How could I ever thank you.
I know the answer, become who I am meant
to be, a healthy human being. Oh, by the way,
since my last appointment, smoking is no longer
a part of me!

Now enough about Jack, let me tell you
about how this seed you planted has grown.
My wife, who looks healthy, young slim, but
her blood work showed she had very high
cholesterol levels. She made the decision to
try my way of eating. Reduced her cholesterol,
feeling better, made the decision to go back
and futher her education, not only did the
seed sprout but a plant is growing. My best
friend complained his legs were killing him, could
not ride motorcycles with us any longer. His doctor
said it is a side effect from his medication,
he offered to change it but with little encouragement
that the effect would not be the same. So he
said, "Well if Jack and his wife are so hyped up
on this new way of eating I will give it a
try also, if they can do it, so can I." Guess
what? He is off the medication that hurt
his legs, next Spring, he will be riding again.
Also they no longer smoke, another one of

Letter to Dr. Patel from her patient - Page 3

④

secretaries at work, has join us in smoking
is not a part of us any longer. This seed you
Dr Petal have planted is really, really growing.
I work in a very high stress job, been doing it
for years. Last Friday around 6 p.m, just as everyone
was leaving the office, problems happened, everything
was falling a part. My boss and I sat down,
I smiled and said let develop a solution. He was
freaking out but we sat there, within about 30
minutes a plan was formulated, problem solved
and we went home for the weekend. The next
Monday my boss asked, what did the VA prescibed
that kept you calm, I need to get some from
my doctor. Now understand my boss is not over weight
but he takes 5 different blood pressure medications
daily and he is 65. I told him that my
physian did not prescribe anything, she taught me
how to eat correctly and how to breathe.
He has started the breathing and claims he feels
better but is pretty resistence on his way
of eating. I will find a way to help motivate
him to change. I think because he is not over
weight he feels he is eating correctly so weigh
loss is not a factor here. But I will find
a way I just need to research.
     So what I am trying to espress in this
letter Dr Patel is not so much that you

Letter to Dr. Patel from her patient - Page 4

(5)

Are healing me, you are also healing others you don't even know, others you have never met. It is my belief, my hope, my mission to take this seed you have planted and not see a plant grow but see a forest grow.

In closing I want to give you my thoughts on the biggest battle we face. Consumerism, I have notice that most commercials are selling products, food, which are bad for us. They put a healthy, beautiful girl. and show her eating a burger with bacon, cheese, chicken, whatever else they can put between 2 buns, with a caloric intake double that of what a body needs plus a list of chemical additives we don't see, leaving the impression, this lady eats it, looks healthy, we will be too. The truth being, we want to make money, she really exercises, never eats this crap but you as consumers don't realize this. This is the same tactic smokers get when cigarette companies could advertise. I watched a Tedx vedio by Dr. Michael Greger, very enlighting.

I want to thank you so very much Dr. Patel, for changing my life and putting me on the road to healing. Your approach could save

Letter to Dr. Patel from her patient - Page 5

⑥

numerous vets and others. Grow the forest,
plant seeds. I will continue on the road
to becoming, healthy, enlightened a living testament
to your practice. Again please share this, you
know it is true, share my medical files I don't
care, I want to help the forest grow. I look
forward to my next lab and appointment because
the path I am on, my prescriptions will be
apart of my PAST. Thank you so very much, reach
out to me anytime. I look forward to our
next visit and please Happy Holidays!!

Letter to Dr. Patel from her patient - Page 6

So, Lifestyle Is Medicine.

And, I am the doctor of the future, now.

———————◦○◦———————

For my Parents, my heart, and my loves.

———————◦○◦———————

About Dr. Karmi Patel, MD, FACP, DipABLM

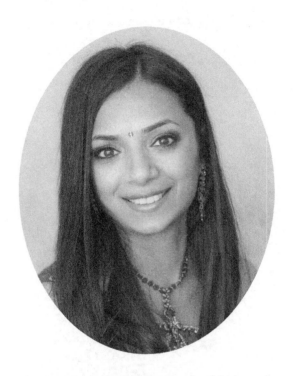

Dr. Karmi Patel is a practicing physician, double board certified in Internal Medicine and Lifestyle Medicine. She received her undergraduate degree from the Pennsylvania State University. Dr. Patel attended Ross University School of Medicine in Dominica and received her medical degree in 2000. She did her residency at St. Peter's University Hospital in New Brunswick, NJ, continuing to serve as chief resident and teaching attending after her training, and was recognized as the recipient of the Sister Marie de Pazzi, CSJP Outstanding Resident Award during her senior year. She currently practices at William C. Tallent VA Outpatient Clinic in Knoxville, TN. Dr. Patel has been part of the American College of Lifestyle Medicine and the Indian Society of Lifestyle Medicine. In addition, she served as Secretary for the American College of Lifestyle Medicine's Veterans Affairs and Dept of Defense Member Interest. Dr. Patel grew up in India and was exposed to herbal medicine with Ayurvedic practice which led to her interest in implementing a whole food plant-based approach for treating, preventing, and reversing diseases. Dr. Patel is a firm believer in the true Hippocrates oath, "Let food be thy medicine and medicine be thy food."

Instagram: https://www.instagram.com/karmipatelmd/

Twitter: https://twitter.com/karmipatelmd

Watch an interview with the co-author:

Co-Author spotlight
DR. KARMI PATEL

Scan Me

21

A Journey of Hope: From Burnout to Blessings, How Lifestyle Medicine Saved Me

Gouri Pimputkar, DO, FACOOG, DipABLM

"You can't go back and change the beginning, but you can start where you are and change the ending."
— C.S. Lewis

I don't recall if there was a defining moment that made me change. All I know is that I could not continue down the same path. There were so many times that my health took a backseat to the continued imbalance of work and life. The irony of the whole situation was that I was supposed to be the one promoting a healthier lifestyle for others. I was supposed to give advice on diet and nutrition for women during adolescence, reproductive years, and menopause. The truth was there were many times that I felt like a fraud.

My personal journey and unhealthy relationship with food and exercise began during my teenage years. Somewhere along the way, on my quest for perfection and acceptance, I learned that food (and later exercise) was the perfect buffer for discomfort. The discomfort was subtle; sometimes, it came in the form of a bad grade on a test, and other times, it was blatant rejection or discrimination. Regardless, I never developed the coping skills to lean into the discomfort but rather did everything in my power to make it disappear . . . quickly. As the years went by, I became embroiled in the rituals of practicing medicine as an OBGYN physician and learned more maladaptive behaviors that would continue to buffer the stress of trying to balance work and family life.

While my story is not unique for overachievers, I was so deep in this reality that I began to wear it like a badge of honor. I suffered in silence with infertility and miscarriages for many years and would rub salt in my wounds by having to put a smile on my face and take care of pregnant women daily. Instead of embracing the trauma, I pushed through it and continued to overwork and numb the pain. While most people embarked on the infertility journey with fierce determination, I found myself "fitting" in my treatments during my busy day. I would never dream of this type of schedule for my patient, yet somehow, it was totally acceptable to me.

Eventually, we were blessed with our children, but the stress of work and now family life took on a new form. My friends and family were in awe of how I was able to manage ALL the things, work many sleepless nights and then go on to plan the perfect kids' birthday party. I took the accolades that were thrown at me as an accomplishment rather than the truth . . . that my overloaded schedule was slowly chipping away at my physical and mental health. The endless electronic medical charting that needed to be completed at the end of the day felt better with mindless grazing of usually healthy snacks. Buffering with Netflix was easier than managing my mind about what was really going on. To compensate for mindless eating, I would over-exercise at ridiculous times in the morning. I would often sacrifice sleep in order to stay on top of my game. I found myself micromanaging my kids and husband in order to stay in control of what I was truly feeling. On the outside, I looked like I had the "perfect" life. I had achieved it all; the career, the beautiful family, a loving husband, great friends, and living in the right neighborhood. On the inside, I was slowly falling apart, piece by piece.

Slowly, I developed insulin resistance, borderline diabetes, elevated cholesterol, auto-immune thyroid disease, and gastrointestinal reflux, even though I looked healthy on the outside. Initially, I was very regimented with diet and exercise. As with anything, if I worked hard enough, I was certain I could beat my fate. Unfortunately, that was not enough because of the constant stress and lack of sleep in the background. I tried every diet and healthy way of living. Subconsciously, I began to chase a number on the scale or a lab value to announce to the world that I had finally arrived "there." I was certain that if I accomplished this, I could finally relax and breathe a bit easier. From counting points or macros to CrossFit and HIIT workouts, the inevitable need for medication to manage my chronic conditions prevailed.

This new way of living was exhausting. I felt like I was continuously running on the hamster wheel of my life. Work, stress, lack of sleep, kids, diet, exercise . . . rinse and repeat; the cycle never seemed to end. Then, the COVID-19 pandemic happened. Alongside modern healthcare experiencing a crisis like never before, our perfect "bubble" was about to burst. Through circumstances both purposeful and unforeseen, we decided to make a cross-country move for my husband's career and work-life balance. We left family and familiarity in order to better our lives. It was the ultimate sacrifice; I would give up what was comfortable in order to improve our family life. As with any move, there were challenges. However, as the dust settled, everyone seemed to acclimate to our new world, everyone except me. I could no longer hide behind the facade of my previous life as evidence that I could make it work.

I found Lifestyle Medicine (LM) by accident. It started with a podcast about managing your health with managing your mind. The message was clear; there was no quick fix or perfect diet to achieve the health goals that I was always striving for. It was all about putting yourself first and approaching your life from a place of love and abundance. THIS was mind-blowing. Never, in all the years of my adult life, did I put myself as a priority and truly practice acts of self-care. Slowly, I started noticing how my body felt with certain foods that I ate. If it didn't feel good, I would no longer indulge in it. Gradually, I moved to a primarily whole food plant-based diet. With that change, the next logical step was to reduce processed flour and sugar. The results were subtle yet utterly profound. The reflux, brain fog, and hot flashes of perimenopause almost disappeared. I felt like I had discovered an ancient secret and could not wait to share it with others.

I began incorporating LM concepts of a WFPBD, exercise and movement, stress management, the importance of sleep, and decreasing risky substances with my patients. As an OBGYN, I treat women through all phases of life. It was empowering to educate teens and adolescents about Lifestyle Medicine. If I had been exposed to these concepts at an early age, maybe my health trajectory would have been different. As for my patients struggling with PCOS and infertility, subtle changes were dramatically changing their lives. Slowly, I had patients that were spontaneously getting pregnant despite years of expensive infertility treatments.

One patient, in particular, lost over 30 lbs in eight months and spontaneously conceived after years of invasive IVF treatments. Her husband was so moved by her transformation that he also adopted a WFPB diet and supported his wife on her journey. When they found out they were pregnant, they had tears in their eyes and told me that I was the first doctor that truly listened and gave them the courage to find another way to make their dreams come true. For my menopausal patients, this concept was a welcomed respite instead of the traditional dependence on hormonal therapy as the only form of treatment. We live in a culture where it is easy to blame "our hormones" for the normal female aging process. Far too often, women become victims to this mindset and give away their power. Many patients believe that weight gain and hot flashes are inevitable, and there are only two choices for relief; suffer in silence or take medications that carry inherent risks (and benefits). By introducing the concepts of a WFPB diet and other LM strategies, many patients decreased their insulin resistance and chronic inflammatory states, which, in turn, improved their transition during the menopausal period. It was always natural for me to meet my patients where they were on their own health journey and provide guidance in a way that had been lost over the years. For the first time in a long time, I finally felt like I had arrived.

The last part of this story is the hardest. While my dependence on medications to manage my chronic diseases was declining, I still had work to do on my mind and stress management. I finally understood that there is no such thing as work-life balance. There are simply certain times of your life when things need more love and attention compared to other times.

It was time to pay attention to myself. The "balance" naturally has started to fall in place. Instead of exercising as a form of punishment or stress relief, I started moving as an act of self-care. I traded my hard-core cardio workouts for walking, yoga, strength training, and simply playing with my children. Managing my stress is an ongoing process. I have learned that progress speaks volumes over perfection. If nothing else, I am sharing my progress with my children so that they can start learning how to manage their minds at an early age and live their best life.

In December 2022, I became board certified in Lifestyle Medicine. I left the traditional practice of Obstetrics and Gynecology to incorporate Lifestyle Medicine concepts into women's health. Instead of the knee-jerk reaction of prescribing medications for illnesses that plague women, I ask the question as to how she got there in the first place. I have achieved personal and professional fulfillment in ways that were previously unimaginable. My impact on healthcare is taking a new direction, and I could not be more excited. As it turns out, Lifestyle Medicine truly saved me.

This chapter is dedicated to the loves of my life. Thank you to my husband and children for giving me the strength, ever-lasting support, and courage to start this new journey. Thank you to my parents, my brother, and his family for always believing in me and inspiring me to be better.

About Dr. Gouri Pimputkar, DO, FACOOG, DipABLM

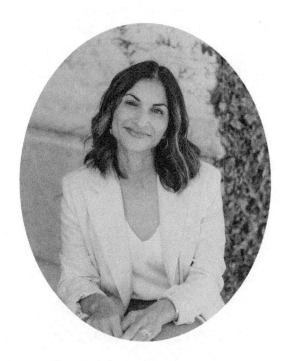

Dr. Gouri Pimputkar is a board-certified Obstetrician and Gynecologist as well as board certified in Lifestyle Medicine. With a strong emphasis on women's health and well-being, Dr. Pimputkar understands the unique needs and challenges women face at every stage of life.

As a trusted advocate, Dr. Pimputkar completed her medical school education at the Arizona College of Osteopathic Medicine and pursued her residency in OBGYN through Ascension Healthcare Systems in Detroit, Michigan. Now residing in sunny central Florida, she cherishes an active lifestyle with her three children, supportive husband, and her beloved Bernedoodle.

Passionate about delivering meaningful health solutions, Dr. Pimputkar combines her expertise in evidence-based gynecology with the transformative principles of Lifestyle Medicine. Her holistic approach addresses a broad range of women's health concerns, including conditions such as PCOS, infertility, metabolic syndrome, and menopause.

Dr. Pimputkar's unique approach to chronic hormonal conditions extends beyond the medical realm, and she inspires women of all ages to take control of their health journey. She nurtures her own well-being by exploring her passions in culinary medicine, yoga, tennis, and mindful meditation. Her commitment to a balanced lifestyle resonates with her patients and empowers them to achieve their best lives.

Website: www.allarahealth.com

Instagram: www.instagram.com/wellnesswithdrgouri/

Watch an interview with the co-author:

Co-Author spotlight
DR. GOURI PIMPUTKAR

22

From Loss to Life: Surprise Blessings and the Benefits of Lifestyle Medicine

Shilpi Pradhan, MD, DipABLM

"The greatest reward of life is the power to do good."
— Dr. Elizabeth Blackwell

We sat down for dinner, and I felt "it." "An elephant sitting on your chest." I had heard this phrase many times in medical school, but it never made sense. But that's exactly what it felt like, such intense, crushing pressure. I couldn't catch my breath. I told my husband, but he was busy getting our kids fed and back to the hotel. We had flown down to Orlando that morning, landing around 10 am, and spent all day at Disney, toting the kids around to the rides. We had finally checked into the hotel, unloaded the car, and headed to dinner. Here we were, just sitting down and trying to relax for the first time, and I was having unbearable pain in my chest. It subsided after about five minutes, and I was grateful. I almost wished I had imagined it. I brushed it off. We finished dinner and headed back to the hotel.

As we were getting ready to go to bed, it started again. I lay down, waiting for the elephant to get off my chest. It wouldn't go anywhere. I tried to close my eyes, but this horrible dread overcame me. I thought, if I go to sleep here tonight, I will not wake up tomorrow morning. I just couldn't shake the feeling. I got up and told my husband. He brushed me off, saying the kids were sleeping and I should go back to sleep. I just couldn't. I got the keys to the rental car and drove myself to the nearest ER, and checked myself in with chest pain. They rushed me back through triage once I said "chest pain." After bloodwork and an EKG, I lay in a trauma bay for two to three hours with a curtain between the next patient and myself. I was in so much pain, but the ER was busy that night, and I didn't need the most help. I just kept crying and praying to get back to my babies. The elephant wouldn't leave me for hours that night.

After a long night listening to the beeping sounds of the monitors in the ER, I was moved to the cardiac monitoring unit in the early morning hours. The other patient in my two-patient room was a much older gentleman who probably also came in for chest pain. The nurses and doctors were kind and told me that my cardiac labs were normal and reassured me that I had not suffered a heart attack. They whisked me off for a cardiac stress test and an echocardiogram the same morning. All of these tests also came back as normal. I drove back to the hotel just in time to arrange lunch for the kids. My husband was anxious and worried about me and our children, and I was exhausted after a long night in the hospital. We both breathed a sigh of relief. We survived the long weekend and made it back home safely to Virginia. I vowed to change my diet. I remembered the risk factors for heart disease from medical school, and my main one was an unhealthy diet full of fried and processed food. I also remembered women having different symptoms of a heart attack, including nausea, vomiting, and stomach pain. I promised myself to get healthier and reduce my risk of heart disease. The episode was a wake-up call to pay attention to my health and diet. I never wanted the stress of feeling like an elephant was sitting on my chest or to worry about my heart health again.

Loss, Infertility, and Surprise Blessings

Since my teenage years, I recall being heartbroken as several doctors told me I might never have children due to a diagnosis of polycystic ovarian syndrome (PCOS). I had little choice other than to believe them. Then, during my fellowship training, I had a surprise pregnancy that turned our worlds upside down with joy and excruciating pain. I experienced the devastating loss of twins due to preterm labor (at 21 weeks of gestation) at the age of 30. This loss, with significant hormone shifts, led to bilateral DeQuervain's tendonitis in both wrists. That year was painful for my body and soul as I finished my fellowship in bilateral wrist braces and cried myself to sleep for months, curled up around the wooden urn of my twins. The loss of our twins and the stress of infertility from PCOS weighed heavily on me. It made me feel like a failure as a woman. I also worried about being a good surgeon after needing bilateral wrist surgery that year. As a coping mechanism, I took time off, took my oral board exam for Ophthalmology, and signed papers to establish an endowed scholarship in the name of our twins. Despite our student loans, we needed a way for our twins to live on and hopefully benefit others through the scholarship. It was the only way I knew how to cope with my grief. And I cried a lot but pretended everything was okay to hide the pain and allow the world to go on.

I've been pregnant five times now, and we are blessed with four children. With all of my pregnancies, I experienced symptoms of preterm labor, although I didn't know exactly what that meant with my twins' pregnancy. After the loss of our twins, I lived in fear of loss again and again. My fear tempered the joys of pregnancy. My second and third pregnancies resulted in two healthy children under the careful watch of a high-risk OB doctor and with medications, daily shots, and bed rest. Through my reading and literature search, I discovered gluten intolerance can contribute to miscarriage, and being gluten-free helped my contractions and preterm labor symptoms. I thought that gluten mainly affected me during pregnancy, so six months postpartum, I returned to eating everything, including gluten-containing food. Only when I had trouble conceiving and needed fertility medications with my third pregnancy did I realize that my infertility was related to not being strictly gluten-free. My research had also taught me gluten intolerance can cause infertility, but it didn't dawn on me back then until after I became gluten-free for that pregnancy. I still didn't realize that gluten affected me outside of pregnancy until that fateful episode of chest pain. I share my story to highlight the fact that with the help of dietary changes, healthy pregnancy is possible for women suffering from PCOS.

Gluten Intolerance

I knew that gluten-containing food in my diet was affecting my health. I was experiencing progressively worsening gluten intolerance leading to dizziness, nausea, diarrhea, intermittent stomach pain, and brain fog. There were times when I was so dizzy I didn't think I could drive to work, but somehow I struggled through it and worked full days. I would have waves of nausea and dizziness when I felt the need to lie down on the floor in the spare room in between seeing patients in my clinic. I always seemed to be sick with a cold, even when my kids were healthy. I was also experiencing similar symptoms with lotions and dry shampoo hair products with wheat in them, which was surprising. Gluten intolerance can range from mild to severe, such as Celiac disease. Gluten in an intolerant patient's diet can also lead to inflammation in different parts of the body, including joints. That inflammation was spreading through my body and causing more than stomach pain. It was slowly taking away the joy of living a normal life. My body felt so weak and like it was aging rapidly. Despite the ongoing symptoms of gluten intolerance, I knew the chest pain that took me to the ER was an entirely different kind of pain. Pain that I never wanted to feel again. Thus, I took the first step and eliminated gluten from my diet permanently.

Learning about Lifestyle Medicine

I decided to learn more about the science of nutrition and its effect on health. It had been a long time since medical school, and perhaps some things were different now. While chatting with a physician colleague, I was gifted the book *Beat the Heart Attack Gene*. Halfway through the book, I learned about Dr. T. Colin Campbell and his online course on Plant-Based Medicine, available at Cornell University. I enrolled, taking a leap of faith that it had the information I needed to help my health. I was a little nervous as I'd never taken an online course like this before with assignments and due dates. I learned about the science, politics, and marketing of food and its influence on dietary patterns and consumer behavior. Learning about camera tricks used by commercials to make food appear more appealing, like glue to make cheese look stretchy, was eye-opening. I was overwhelmed to learn about the sea's dead zones from pollution and overfishing, and the dredging of the ocean floor. The harmful environmental effects of cattle farming and meat production from deforestation for animal agriculture and the harmful effects of their waste products made me sad. I wanted everyone to take this course and learn what I was learning. The course discussed lobbying in the food industry to allow continued sales and marketing of unsafe products like processed meat (classified as a carcinogen by the World Health Organization) and the politics of what is included on the plate of a student's school lunch. I learned to identify medical studies sponsored by the food industry and to look at the fine print of studies. I absorbed knowledge from the giants in Lifestyle Medicine, such as Dr. T. Colin Campbell, Dr. Caldwell Esselstyn, Dr. Dean Ornish, Dr. Neal Barnard, Dr. Michael Gregor, and many others. After listening to the health benefits of plants and vegetables, I learned about this new field of Lifestyle Medicine and went vegan for the first time.

My New Diet

Being plant-based, gluten-free, and vegan was hard, but my body loved it. Even my family wondered what I was going to eat! I felt more energetic, and I didn't get sick as often. My family was initially skeptical of my new diet, but they supported me and ate the food I made based on recipes from our newly purchased vegan cookbooks. I watched documentaries like *Forks over Knives* and *Game Changers* with my children. I wanted to educate them on everything I had learned about nutrition and health.

My menstrual cycles became more regular within three months of my new diet. And thankfully, I have not had another episode of chest pain.

Surprisingly, with my dietary changes, I became pregnant again at age 40 without trying. It was a total shock to me and my whole family. I didn't realize my improved fertility resulted from a plant-based diet which helped regulate my PCOS, until I became pregnant again for the fifth time at 42 years old. My last two pregnancies were considered "geriatric pregnancies," and I was considered "advanced maternal age," leading to gestational high blood pressure. The side effects of high blood pressure were scary, including loss of hearing (due to fluid in my inner ear) and facial numbness. Finally, worsening headaches led to semi-urgent C-sections for one of these pregnancies. Thankfully, my high blood pressure and other symptoms resolved with delivery. Despite these issues, these pregnancies felt less stressful with fewer contractions, likely because of my dietary changes, even though I was in my 40s now. Pressured not to be vegan during my pregnancies, I could still have full-term healthy babies by being gluten-free and increasing whole foods, and eating a more plant-forward diet.

I found similar stories in Dr. Barnard's latest book, _Your Body In Balance_, of improved fertility and regulated hormones with a whole food plant-based (WFPB) diet. Veganism and being gluten-free helped regulate my hormones, PCOS, and menstrual cycles so much that everything was like clockwork, and we got pregnant without trying, TWICE! That's how much the field of Lifestyle Medicine has impacted me. LM has given me two beautiful surprise children to add to my brood; we now have four children.

Lifestyle Medicine has given me the gift of life and hope. It has given my family an alternative way of looking at food and shifted our standard meals. Indians are generally either vegetarian or "chickaterian," or people who consume chicken and fish as part of their diet. Indian families tend to consume a lot of dairy products such as milk, yogurt, buttermilk, and fried food items. They also use butter or ghee (clarified butter) to prepare homemade sweets. Indian Americans sometimes follow the Standard American Diet (SAD) and eat beef, pork, lamb, and goat meat in addition to chicken and seafood. My family had also adopted the SAD. However, with the help of my LM knowledge, I convinced our family to go back to a "chickaterian" diet, and many days are vegan meal days, as we embrace Suzy Cameron's diet of One Meal a Day (*The OMD Plan* book) to help save ourselves and our environment.

Getting Certified

I decided to take the Lifestyle Medicine board exam in 2020 during the COVID-19 pandemic and passed to become officially board-certified. Despite having an infant, we had time off from work because of the pandemic. I had an incredible group of physician colleagues to study with for three months, almost daily, on Zoom. Together as a group, we have improved our health and the health of our families. We developed strong social bonds by studying for the exam, sharing life stories, recipes, and much more. We have all benefited from our group, not only in our health but also in building our community. These friendships are hard to foster as we age, but they were made possible through LM, Facebook, and Zoom. Many of these dear friends are co-authors of this book.

How Lifestyle Medicine Affects My Ophthalmology Practice

As an Ophthalmologist, LM has even impacted how I counsel my patients with diabetes about the care of their eyes. I introduce the WFPB diet and urge them to add greens to their daily meals. I reorient the conversation with patients who have suffered a stroke and other cardiovascular events and those experiencing visual field damage towards learning about how their current diets could contribute to their illness and vision loss. I'm also helping change the trajectory of a few patients' inflammatory eye disease. In particular, I unknowingly convinced one of my patients suffering from nodular scleritis from rheumatoid arthritis to become vegan with my LM discussions. Despite being on oral steroids, she lost 60 pounds in three months (prednisone can cause weight gain). With these dietary modifications, she hasn't experienced a flare-up of her eye disease in many years. I believe the change in her diet helped control her eye disease, in addition to her medications. She has convinced her family members, including her grandchildren, to adopt a more plant-forward diet and brags about her grandkids making kale chips and salads when she comes for a visit.

Among patients suffering from ankylosing spondylitis, I help reduce recurrent iritis by eliminating gluten from their diet (gluten is linked to uveitis). I regularly counsel my patients with dry eyes about the importance of a plant-forward diet and other LM factors, such as sleep which can affect dry eye disease. In my recently published book, *Goodbye, Dry Eye!* I have written about how diet and other LM factors affect dry eye disease. I educate patients with macular degeneration on the benefits of Age-Related Eye Disease Study (AREDS2) supplements per the National Institutes of Health (NIH) guidelines. In addition, I talk about the beneficial effects of whole foods (not processed), particularly kale (which has a high content of lutein and zeaxanthin — essential nutrients for the photoreceptors in our retina). I urge smoking cessation in patients with glaucoma and macular degeneration because it is a known risk factor for the progression of these diseases.

Anyone who asks me questions about supplements or nutrition in the clinic now gets a quick introduction to LM, the benefits of eating whole foods, being plant-based, and avoiding beef and pork. If they ask for more, I direct them to my website, where I have links to my favorite LM books and links/resources to other doctors who have dedicated their lives to Lifestyle Medicine. Initially, patients would get a 30-minute discussion about LM (after my board certification), and I would get behind in my schedule, but now I've tapered that down to 5 minutes. However, I'm just as enthusiastic about the field of LM. Seeing my journey, a few patients have found the courage to have children in their 40s after seeing me have my last two children. It's gratifying and simply amazing that I was able to help these women further their dreams of their own families. I'm humbled to know that there are more humans in the world because of my pregnancy history and because of LM's impact on my fertility.

Conclusion

Lifestyle Medicine is the future of medicine. Lifestyle Medicine has given us the tools and the knowledge to live sustainably and lead healthier lives by growing and consuming food that preserves our planet for future generations. We must change our medical model to wellness and prevention, keeping the six pillars of health from LM in focus. These changes will enable us to live healthy lives, prevent disease in ourselves and future generations, and potentially reverse chronic diseases. Lifestyle Medicine is not a cure-all for all conditions but a stepping stone for a healthier version of us, the collective of humanity. We will always need modern medications, research, and the development of new drugs. However, if we can decrease the disease burden among ourselves and the medical system, we can use those healthcare dollars to improve our collective health. By adopting the tools provided by LM, we can be proactive about living healthier, longer, and more meaningful lives. I hope my story and my patients' stories inspire you to take charge of your health.

This chapter is dedicated to my parents, Dr. Shekhar Pradhan and Mrs. Savita Pradhan, the best grandparents to our four children, my husband, Dr. Kumar Abhishek, the best father to our kids, and my children (Shreya, Ankit, Asha, and Priya) for making me a mother.

Thank you, God, for all the blessings and opportunities in my life.

Thank you to my co-authors for trusting me to share their amazing and personal stories in this book.

References:

Bale, B., & Doneen, A. (2014b). *Beat the Heart Attack Gene: The Revolutionary Plan to Prevent Heart Disease, Stroke, and Diabetes*. Turner Publishing Company.

Plant-Based Nutrition. eCornell. https://ecornell.cornell.edu/certificates/nutrition/plant-based-nutrition/.

Barnard, N. D. (2020). *Your body in balance: The New Science of Food, Hormones, and Health*. Hachette UK.

Cameron, S. A. (2019). *The OMD Plan: Swap One Meal a Day to Save Your Health and Save the Planet*. Atria Books.

Favorite Lifestyle Medicine Resources: https://www.eyedoctormd.org/lifestyle-medicine/

Favorite Cookbooks Listed on my website:

https://www.eyedoctormd.org/health-corner/lifestyle-medicine-cookbooks-and-blogs/

Other books by Dr. Pradhan

Pradhan, S. (2023). *Goodbye, Dry Eye! Expert advice on remedies and relief for dry eyes*. Pradhan Publications LLC. https://amzn.to/3Jnn7Bk including a Lifestyle Medicine section.

Please read the Introduction in this book, also written by Dr. Pradhan.

About Dr. Shilpi Pradhan, MD, DipABLM

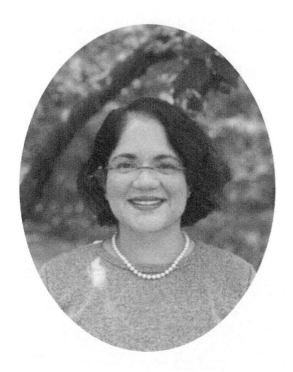

Dr. Shilpi Pradhan is a board-certified Ophthalmologist and Lifestyle Medicine doctor, a mother of four beautiful children, and a personal finance and real estate enthusiast. She's interested in the impact Lifestyle Medicine can have on eye diseases and overall health.

Dr. Pradhan went to Emory University, Atlanta, GA, for college and completed medical school at Washington University in St. Louis, Missouri. Her medical training included a transitional residency year at Carilion Clinic in Roanoke, VA, an Ophthalmology residency at the Medical College of Virginia at Virginia Commonwealth University in Richmond, VA, and a Cornea, External Disease, and Refractive Surgery fellowship at the University of Pittsburgh Medical Center in Pittsburgh, PA. She worked as an Assistant Professor at Saint Louis University in St. Louis, MO, in 2012 and loved teaching residents before moving to Virginia.

She has owned her solo private practice, Eye Doctor MD PC in Glen Allen, Virginia, since 2015, and practices Ophthalmology and also provides education in Lifestyle Medicine to her patients. She has also completed the Plant-Based Nutrition Certificate from eCornell and the T. Colin Campbell Center for Nutrition Studies in 2019.

To honor the memory of their twins, Dr. Pradhan and her husband, Dr. Abhishek, established an endowed scholarship in their name, called the *Twin Angels Abhishek Pradhan Scholarship*, at Washington University in St. Louis School of Medicine in 2009, and it has been distributed annually since 2017.

Website: www.eyedoctormd.org

YouTube: https://www.youtube.com/@dr.shilpipradhan

Instagram: https://instagram.com/drshilpipradhan/

LinkedIn: https://www.linkedin.com/in/shilpi-pradhan-b5306114

Watch an interview with the co-author:

Co-Author spotlight
DR. SHILPI PRADHAN

Scan Me

23

Good Health Begins in the Gut: A Gastroenterologist's Journey in Lifestyle Medicine

Supriya Rao, MD, DipABLM, DipABOM

"The road to health is paved with good intestines."
— Sherry A. Rogers

M s. J was my last patient of a long clinic day. She was referred to me because she was recently diagnosed with fatty liver. As a gastroenterologist, I managed many patients with fatty liver—but my advice was not enough. I would tell people they needed to change their diet and exercise more, then recheck their labs in a few months. Obviously, this prescription was vague and did not help many people. Ms. J said she was already doing the best she could with regard to her health. I was growing tired of not being able to take care of my patients in the way I wanted and knew I had to seek out more education.

I started with the Obesity Medicine (OM) curriculum in 2019 and learned a significant amount about risk factors and contributors to obesity and how to treat it as a chronic disease. This allowed me to start having conversations with my patients about metabolic disease and its relation to gastrointestinal disorders. Fatty liver was my version of heart disease as a GI specialist. I wanted to help people improve their health and lose weight to avoid further progression to inflammation, fibrosis, and, ultimately, cirrhosis. After completing the OM certification, I was able to start an obesity medicine mini-practice within my gastroenterology practice and expand my reach to patients with other chronic medical conditions related to obesity.

While I was seeing success with my patients and they were excited about the changes they were seeing, I was not counseling them effectively enough regarding lifestyle. I had received little nutrition education throughout my training and felt ill-prepared in coaching patients through this. While looking for more resources to help, I stumbled upon the American College of Lifestyle Medicine (ACLM) website. I reviewed the six pillars of health: plant-based nutrition, regular physical activity, stress management, restorative sleep, meaningful social connections, and avoidance of risky substances. This approach to health would be my next step in empowering my patients to make sustainable changes in their lives and promote wellness instead of just treating illness.

I completed the Lifestyle Medicine (LM) board certification and felt better equipped to improve whole person health. I took the knowledge I acquired through the ACLM curriculum to my practice and counseled patients in a more meaningful way. I saw them respond differently and want to take more action to live healthier lives. After every colonoscopy I performed, I spent more time discussing the benefits of a healthy lifestyle on colon cancer risk and colon polyp formation. Irritable Bowel Syndrome (IBS) symptoms can flare up during periods of stress, inactivity, and unhealthy eating. By discussing lifestyle techniques, my patients were better able to take control of their symptoms. I became a health coach through Vanderbilt University because I saw the power of coaching and how it can transform lives through supporting self-empowerment and self-efficacy.

While I was seeing improvements in my one-on-one patient encounters, I couldn't help but feel that I wanted to effect greater change on a broader scale. I wanted to find a program that would be accessible to anyone who needed lifestyle changes. This finally came to fruition when I discovered the Lifestyle Medicine Institute and their course called PIVIO through my colleague. This 18-module course takes place over 12 weeks and explores all the topics of LM and adds in the critical aspect of behavior change and habit making, all while in a group led by me. This program has been transformative for patients, from discussing optimal eating, activity, and rest to mastering motivation, building relationships, and habit hacking. With PIVIO, we can deliver care to a wider base of patients and have it be accessible to all as it is covered by insurance. This has been a game changer in giving patients the time and space to discuss their medical conditions, lifestyle habits, and behavioral barriers. They also have a built-in support system and are able to bounce ideas off the other participants. We have had dozens of patients go through the PIVIO program with great success. Patients have had significant improvements in weight, biometrics, and labs, such as cholesterol and hemoglobin A1c. It has been a humbling and gratifying experience to offer this program to our community, and I hope that it continues to grow.

With all of these exciting developments going on at work, I also made several changes at home. I have been a vegetarian my entire life but did not always follow a whole food diet. I also had typical processed foods in my diet, so I wanted to work on changing that. Exercise and improved sleep quality also became a priority.

My husband is also a gastroenterologist and was fully on board with lifestyle changes. We discuss gastrointestinal conditions and the gut microbiome at home with our children. The gut microbiome project states that we must have 30 unique plants in our diet to ensure healthy microbiome diversity and overall health. We often count the number of plants at each meal. My children are interested in where their food comes from and want to take part in cooking meals. It's been rewarding to talk about what a healthy lifestyle entails and how we can make small sustainable changes in our modern lives to achieve that goal.

Lifestyle Medicine has been instrumental in transforming the health of my patients and my family. It has taught me that it is possible to prevent and even reverse chronic disease with a healthy lifestyle transformation and that focusing on whole person health is a necessity. The way I practice medicine has shifted dramatically over the years, and I find myself discussing lifestyle and behavior change more and more with patients and colleagues. I am hopeful that this will be where the field of medicine is going, and excited to spread the word that lifestyle medicine truly heals.

This chapter is dedicated to my loving parents and siblings, as well as my ever-supportive husband and kids. Thank you for being my champions and the reasons I continue this work.

About Dr. Supriya Rao, MD, DipABLM, DipABOM

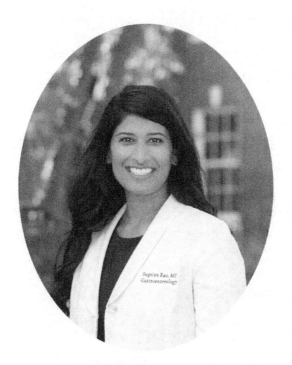

Dr. Supriya Rao is a quadruple board-certified physician in Internal Medicine, Gastroenterology, Obesity Medicine, and Lifestyle Medicine who focuses on digestive disorders, gut health, the microbiome, obesity medicine, and women's health and wellness. She received her undergraduate degree from the Massachusetts Institute of Technology, after which she graduated from Duke University School of Medicine. She completed her internship and residency in Internal Medicine at the Hospital at the University of Pennsylvania. She went on to complete her fellowship in Gastroenterology at Boston Medical Center. She is a managing partner at Integrated Gastroenterology Consultants, located in the greater Boston area. She completed further board certification in Obesity and Lifestyle Medicine and is the Director of Medical Weight Loss at Lowell General Hospital. She also runs the motility program, which focuses on disorders of the esophagus, irritable bowel syndrome, and anorectal conditions.

She is passionate about empowering people to improve their health through sustainable changes in their lifestyle and runs an intensive LM curriculum through her office. She loves to cook and share her passion for plant-based cuisine with her family and friends.

Website- https://www.integratedgic.com/blog/supriya-rao and http://www.gutsygirlmd.com/

Instagram: www.instagram.com/gutsygirlmd

LinkedIn: https://www.linkedin.com/in/supriya-rao-md-dipl-abom-dipablm-b058b791

Watch an interview with the co-author:

Co-Author spotlight
DR. SUPRIYA RAO

Scan Me

24

THE HEALING POWER OF LIFESTYLE MEDICINE

Tatyana Reznik, MD, FACP, DipABLM

"Optimum nutrition is the medicine of tomorrow."
— Linus Pauling (Nobel Prize winner)

Nutrition is my favorite part of Lifestyle Medicine. My introduction to the transformative effects of nutrition started over two decades ago after a brief conversation with a kind stranger.

It was a busy evening in the ER. Our next patient was a young lady who fainted while walking. She was brought in by a bystander who happened to witness her fainting. He carried her in his arms all the way to our hospital. It was not a small distance as our hospital was several blocks away, and it was raining.

I do not know his name, so I remember him as a 'Kind Stranger.' He appeared to be in his mid-40s, with an athletic build, glowing skin, and healthy-looking hair. He radiated kindness, vitality, and strength. The patient's friend, another young lady, was nearby and was providing her history. She kept thanking the Kind Stranger for helping and bringing the patient all the way to the ER.

They were chatting, and somehow he mentioned his age. That caught my attention.

He was 62 years old. Sixty-two?! I thought I misheard, so I asked him directly. Yes, 62!

I asked, surprised, "How is that possible, what is your secret? You look like you are in your mid-40s. What helps you stay young and strong? Are you exercising five hours a day, every day? Good genes?"

He laughed and replied, "Not at all. I seldom exercise, but I have always been physically active at work. Both my parents and grandparents were not that healthy and died before the age of 60. I have just been eating right since I was in my early 20s."

"What do you eat?" both the patient's friend and I asked in unison. I expected to hear about some exotic diet and supplements.

"I only eat plants," he replied. "No animal food at all. Most of my food is fresh, with plenty of greens and salads every day. No processed food, no sodas, and almost no sugar except on special occasions. For dessert and snacks, I eat fruits or nuts. You can try it and see. What also helps is that I don't sweat the small stuff, which keeps my stress levels down."

"But where do you get your protein from?" I asked. He clearly didn't lack muscle mass.

"There is plenty of protein in beans, veggies, and greens. I also love eating buckwheat, so I use it instead of other grains in many meals. It is rich in protein. Vitamin B12 is the only supplement I take on a vegan diet," he shared.

The Kind Stranger added that he became vegan because he loved animals and felt it was unnecessarily cruel to keep eating them. He told us that after replacing animal food with fresh veggies and greens, he noticed an increase in energy, mental clarity, and his skin became clearer. It was a positive "side effect."

He told us that with time, he became more interested in health benefits, read a lot about it, and removed most of the processed food and sugar from his diet, replacing it with extra fruits, berries, and nuts. He noticed that his immunity improved. Now, he hardly ever gets sick with a cold.

I was truly impressed.

He left shortly after, and we were busy with other patients, but I kept thinking about what he had said.

I felt like someone had opened the window and let fresh air in. It was permission, hope, a lighthouse showing the way to health and vitality in the darkness.

The truth is that I had wanted to be vegan since I was a little child because I love animals. I simply didn't want to eat them. There are so many delicious fruits and vegetables to eat. I didn't think at that time about the health improvement whatsoever.

However, everyone around me kept saying, "If you do not eat meat, you will not have enough protein, and you will be weak and sick." So I was scared to change my diet to plant-based. I believed them, and I was afraid to get sick.

Meeting that Kind Stranger and witnessing his health success opened the door for me to do what I always wanted to do. Not only was he not "malnourished, sick, and weak," but he was fine, even better than fine! Witnessing his example was liberating.

The next morning I decided to give a plant-based diet a try for just one month. I thought that since it is such a short period of time, I can try anything for one month. If I do not feel well or miss eating meat and other animal food too much, I can always go back to my previous diet after a month.

One month passed, and I actually felt fine. I initially missed the taste of cheese, ice cream, and fish but didn't want to go back to eating animal food. So I stayed on a vegan diet for another month and then a third. Then it became my usual way of eating. Several months later, I stopped craving any animal products.

I had completed training in nursing school prior to medical school. At the time of that event, I was working nights in the ER as a nurse, doing 16-hour shifts every third night while studying in medical school during the daytime. I was routinely sleep-deprived. Life was very busy, and I often didn't have time to rest.

The unexpected outcome that I quickly noticed during the first month after eliminating animal food was that I was surprisingly not as tired as I used to be. Somehow, I had more energy and could think clearly without getting too sleepy during the day after my night shifts. I was often able to maintain alertness even without coffee! This increase in energy encouraged me to continue this way of eating.

Years passed, and I graduated from medical school, then completed additional training and became a Cardiologist. I noticed that when I first met most of our patients, they ate unhealthy and processed food. I always tried to share what I had learned about a plant-based diet to help them not only with medications but also with a lifestyle change, so they can have long-lasting benefits.

I later immigrated to the US in 2001, completed Internal Medicine residency training, and started working as a hospitalist physician at a hospital. I was surprised and even shocked by both the large number of patients with obesity-related illnesses and the high cost of medical bills in the US. It prompted me to read more about nutrition and various other ways to preserve one's health.

I made a goal to find out as much as possible about how lifestyle can improve health. I read numerous articles, blogs, and books, watched documentaries, and joined plant-based Facebook groups, exchanging plant-based recipes and ideas. I found it really fascinating how sometimes our body can heal itself if the correct lifestyle changes are made. I made sure to share my knowledge with my patients.

Many years later, I still continued on a plant-based diet. I was at my perfect weight and felt great. I was cooking and meal-prepping at home and enjoyed experimenting with creating various new salads and soups. Being a busy physician mom with limited free time, I especially enjoyed creating new recipes for nutritious meals that require very little time to prepare.

After learning about green smoothies, I tried various combinations and came up with many healthy and delicious recipes that I now share with others. When I cooked, I often made several extra portions and froze them so I would always have a healthy meal at home. I also realized that my body is sensitive to gluten, so I tried to avoid it.

Then, the pandemic hit and brought with it a lot of stress. I was working long hours at the hospital, taking care of many patients who were sick with COVID-19. We were often short-staffed. As a hospitalist physician, I often spent 12–16+ hours a day at work. I often had no time or energy left to cook, so I ate whatever was available in the hospital cafeteria, which at that time was often lacking whole food plant-based meals.

What also contributed to my diet change is that one week prior to the start of the COVID-19 lockdown, a pipe in our kitchen had a major leak and caused water damage to the floor in half of the house. We moved to a hotel, then to a rental room, and started the renovation. When the pandemic began, everything became delayed for months. As a result, it took almost a year to complete the renovation and to be able to use our kitchen again.

My diet was vegan but not whole food plant-based anymore. There is a huge difference I didn't realize at that time, and I teach it to people now. This difference is a major reason why some vegan diets fail.

Whole food plant-based diet (WFPBD) means no processed food in addition to vegan food. It means to eat fresh or cooked unprocessed food without preservatives and without excessive sugar. It is also paramount that the majority of food be vegetables and fruits rather than bread and macaroni.

Whole food in my diet was replaced with fried potatoes in the form of French fries, tater tots, chips, or some other processed packaged food.

My weight started climbing up, and my energy levels started falling down. In an attempt to eat something other than fried potatoes and to add proteins, I added eggs, fish, and dairy back into my diet and eventually added all sorts of processed unhealthy snacks.

One day, I noticed that I could no longer fit into any of my clothes. I bought new clothes two sizes larger but eventually, they became too small for me too. I bought bigger clothes again. Finally, I bought a new scale and realized how much extra weight I gained. It explained a lot. I decided to make my health a priority.

I went back to implementing the whole food plant-based diet, which allowed my body to thrive. First, I stopped eating processed, unhealthy snacks and added almonds, walnuts, and cashews instead. I added large salads and greens as my meals at least once a day, each and every day. I made several other changes. Desserts became fresh fruits and berries rather than cakes and ice cream. I also added intermittent fasting, a technique used in obesity medicine to improve metabolism.

After shedding 31 pounds, I felt better. And an unexpected thing happened—the hot flashes which had frequently interfered with my life last year became manageable within two months into this diet, and now, are almost gone. My quality of life improved significantly.

I love learning about various ways to improve health and found the annual Lifestyle Medicine conference by the American College of Lifestyle Medicine (ACLM). I signed up to attend out of curiosity.

During that conference, I discovered evidence-based data supporting the positive effects of various lifestyle medicine interventions on chronic disease. I already knew from practical experience and from multiple other sources that nutrition and other lifestyle interventions work in general, but now I was equipped with the data from scientific research behind it.

I learned that Lifestyle Medicine interventions not only can prevent but sometimes also can improve and even reverse some chronic illnesses, such as cardiovascular diseases, type 2 diabetes, obesity, and more.

After attending a Lifestyle Medicine conference, I decided to obtain more skills and knowledge about simple but effective tools that nutrition and other lifestyle medicine pillars of health provide so that I can help my patients better. I became a member of the ACLM and immersed myself in learning from the various resources they offer.

In addition to nutrition, I learned about and started practicing meditation and other mindfulness tools, which can de-stress a busy life. These tools helped improve my general well-being. I learned various ways to manage stress and add more joy into a person's life, and now I help others follow the same path.

I completed additional training, passed an exam, became a Certified Life Coach, and even launched a podcast called *Voices of Women Physicians*. Healthy nutrition has helped me have energy for the many projects I enjoy doing.

After learning as much as I could about various evidence-based interventions, I passed an exam and became board certified in Lifestyle Medicine.

Now, following the principles of Lifestyle Medicine has not only become part of my life, but it has also become part of what I use to help my family, friends, patients, and anyone who asks about additional ways to improve their health.

I believe Lifestyle Medicine has huge potential and offers effective solutions that I wish everyone knew about. I made Lifestyle Medicine counseling a part of my routine conversations with my patients. I also share helpful information about Lifestyle Medicine and the WFPB diet,

including links, resources, and recipes on my website with anyone interested in improving and preserving their health.

━━━◆○◆━━━

*Acknowledgment: Many thanks to
my daughter, Elena Rabinovich, for
her help in editing my chapter.*

━━━◆○◆━━━

About Dr. Tatyana Reznik, MD, FACP, DipABLM

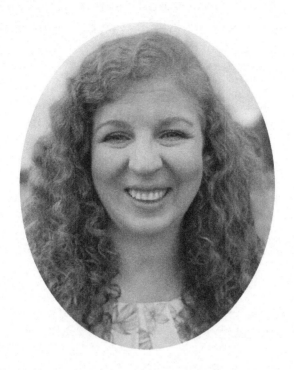

Dr. Tatyana Reznik is a practicing physician with over 25 years of clinical experience. She is double board-certified in Internal Medicine and Lifestyle Medicine, a mother, a Certified Life Coach, the host of the Voices of Women Physicians Podcast, and an author. She immigrated to the US over 20 years ago from Uzbekistan where she was a practicing Cardiologist.

In the US, she completed residency training at the University of Nevada, Reno, and has been practicing Hospital Medicine in California since then. She is passionate about helping people improve their health and well-being.

In her coaching practice, she helps professional women turn their dreams and ideas into reality. Through the combination of mindset shifts as well as practical tips and resources, she helps them leave behind overwhelm and self-doubt and create a joyful life.

Dr. Reznik hosts the *Voices of Women Physicians* Podcast, where she interviews women physician experts, leaders, and innovators who share their inspiring journeys and helpful practical tips from their areas of expertise in and outside of medicine.

Her Facebook group, *Voices of Women Physicians,* is a community of women physicians where they share helpful practical tips to make busy life easier and more joyful.

Dr. Reznik co-authored the upcoming new book, AI in Medicine.

In her free time, Dr. Reznik enjoys spending time with family and friends, creating easy and delicious recipes, learning new things, traveling, reading, and photography.

Website: https://www.joyfulsuccessliving.com

Podcast: https://podcasts.apple.com/us/podcast/voices-of-women-ph ysicians/id1630624425

LinkedIn: www.linkedin.com/in/tatyana-reznik-md-facp

Facebook: https://www.facebook.com/tatyana.reznik.16?mibextid=L QQJ4d

Facebook Group:

https://www.facebook.com/groups/190596326343825/?ref=share_gr oup_link&exp=9594

Instagram: https://www.instagram.com/joyfulsuccessliving/

Linktree: https://linktr.ee/joyfulsuccess

Watch an interview with the co-author:

Co-Author spotlight
DR. TATYANA REZNIK

25

WE ARE OUR MOST IMPORTANT PATIENT

Trisha Schimek, MD, MSPH, DipABLM

"Self-care is not selfish or self-indulgent. We cannot nurture others from a dry well. We need to take care of our own needs first, so that we can give from our surplus, our abundance. When we nurture others from a place of fullness, we feel renewed instead of taken advantage of."
— Jennifer Louden

I reached a professional and personal low in 2021 when the world was one year into the COVID-19 pandemic. I was an early career physician with a mission to care for the underserved, and I was pregnant with my second child. For the first year of the pandemic, it was easy to immerse myself into my career, and for over a year and a half, I worked without taking any vacation days. After all, I was healthy and young, and there was plenty of need for doctors. Plus, I was conserving my vacation days for my child's birth because my job did not offer any paid maternity leave. But in the second year of the pandemic, clinic days began to feel monotonous and unfulfilling. Each day, I showed up for my patients and colleagues to listen to them express their feelings of anxiety and despair. However, because of social distancing and long work hours, I stopped seeking support from my friends and colleagues to process my own stress. To make matters worse, being pregnant made it more difficult to recruit my usual coping strategies. Pregnancy-induced nausea made eating carbohydrates more appealing than my normal diet of fruits, vegetables, and beans. Exercising felt like a chore and more draining than usual, and prenatal exercise modifications left me feeling dissatisfied when I could convince myself to work out.

Five years earlier, I had completed a global health fellowship and made the decision to work at a safety-net county health system because it was a domestic position where I would employ my global health background to care for a diverse patient population. Additionally, it offered an opportunity to educate family medicine residents with a similar mission. At the start of my job in 2017 and into the start of the pandemic, the novelty, the mission, and the people were able to sustain the long working days, but eventually, I started to feel ineffective and exhausted. My zest to problem-solve and tackle obstacles dwindled, and I was developing a learned helplessness in a broken system. I was able to show up, function, and attempt to provide excellent care, but my resilience was not enough to handle the workload. Pessimistic thoughts began to replace my usual optimism. I was able to see the dysfunction in the system and the burnout in others, but part of my personality made it hard to admit burnout in myself.

In 2021, I was selected to participate in the American Academy Family Physician Fellowship in Physician Well-being and Leadership. I originally applied, hoping to learn concrete strategies for systemic change, which I could employ to help my colleagues and residents. Ultimately, the result was quite ironic. During that fellowship, I realized my feelings of exhaustion, ineffectiveness, and lack of personal accomplishment were a sign of professional burnout. Continually adding more responsibilities without taking the time to reflect on my experience and values would potentially further my burnout. Thus, I decided to slow down, reflect, and be more intentional in my efforts. As part of that fellowship, I met physicians practicing Lifestyle Medicine (LM), an interprofessional society of health professionals researching and applying evidence-based lifestyle medicine practices for themselves and patients.

As part of my background in public health and global health, I have a deep understanding of the social determinants of health, or what are the structural, environmental, and political forces affecting a population's health. Public health interventions are often multifaceted and can influence large-scale change, but they can also be time-intensive with higher resource and labor costs. While I have more empathy for each of my individual patient's situations, this knowledge left me feeling powerless to the greater societal factors influencing their outcomes. This is where LM equipped me with tools to have effective conversations with patients to promote behavior change that promoted individual health and well-being. These were the tools I needed to implement into my clinic visits.

In 2022, I delved deeper into the field of Lifestyle Medicine and pursued board certification. I learned the six pillars of lifestyle, each of them promoting health and well-being. A deficiency in one of the pillars can have negative consequences on one's health. When I started this journey, I realized I was personally most deficient in stress management and emotional well-being. Previously, I had positively managed stress by eating well, engaging in physical exercise, and socializing with friends and family. Time constraints of motherhood and my busy career had decreased the time and attention I was spending in those areas. Instead of taking time to cook nutritious meals, I started to include more quick, easy, processed food alternatives into my diet. My husband bought "nutritious" snack foods that were "made with vegetables" but were just as processed as potato chips or cookies. For dinner, we heated up prepared frozen meals, but these were packed with sodium and preservatives. Thankfully, I had some old habits and memories of healthy eating and physical exercise that I could rely on once I made a commitment to change. As I learned more about the benefits of adopting a whole food plant-based diet, it convinced me that this diet was the solution for the metabolic disease I was treating daily in the clinic. The irony of our healthcare industry spending billions of dollars on new pharmaceutical therapies when disease could be reversed by radically changing the food we consume and returning to basic whole food nutrition was not lost on me.

As expected, personal change was slow and winding. Just like all human beings, I am influenced by my environment and my loved ones. Therefore, being questioned or doubted by them was sometimes uncomfortable. At times, it was easier to give in to social pressure than to stay true to what I was learning. Humans are tribal creatures and naturally want to belong to a group and not go against the grain. Dairy was the hardest for me to cut out. Like most people, I had believed that yogurt, cheese, and milk were the superior choice for calcium consumption and were all part of many weekly meals—enchiladas, pizza, overnight oats, and breakfast yogurt parfaits. I found inspiration for creating healthier alternatives to my favorite meal by reading vegan food blogs and cookbooks. The internet made it possible to find healthier recipes for old favorites. Fortunately, there were also more plant-based alternative products readily available to explore. For instance, to replace cow milk, now there is soy, almond, oat, flax, or hemp milk. I made it a game to start exploring my options and trying new products. I took care to also read the nutrition labels to avoid replacing a plant-based processed food for another processed food. Throughout all of this, I constantly needed to remind myself that small changes were progress and small setbacks were learning opportunities that did not equate with failure.

That same year, I signed up to participate in my first sprint triathlon. I was five months postpartum when I decided to train and get back into regular fitness. I always loved biking and running, but now I had to learn to swim. There were lots of "firsts" throughout the next few months, buying a racing swimsuit and goggles, finding a training pool, wearing a wetsuit, and training out in open water. Crossing the finish line at eight months postpartum was a wonderful personal accomplishment that motivated me to go on and sign up for future races. Moreover, returning to regular physical activity was such a mental health game changer for me. As a new mom, I had less time to myself, so engaging in a workout by myself was how I engaged in my own self-care.

Of all the pillars, the one that needed the most personal attention and, consequently, has reshaped the way I engage with the world is stress management. As previously illustrated, I noticed that I was allowing daily stressors to pile up and build to chronic stress. A single stressful event or intermittently feeling stressed is not inherently harmful to us as humans. In fact, the right amount of stress can help us act and rise to challenges. The negative impact of stress occurs when we are not responding to or managing life's stressors. When I reflected, I was able to realize that I had many examples of positively confronting and coping with stress during my physician training. However, in 2021 when I was experiencing burnout, I was taking less time to engage in effective stress management and thus started to feel the pileup and internalization of chronic stress. I was most familiar with understanding chronic stress by observing it in my patients who were facing structural violence in the form of racism, financial difficulties, unstable housing, and unemployment, leading to and complicating chronic health conditions. Since I was not experiencing those particular hardships, I had a hard time acknowledging that I could be experiencing chronic stress too.

Scientific research shows that chronic stress leads to persistently elevated cortisol levels which can negatively impact our biological system and fan the fire of chronic illness and worsen mental health. When I finally stopped to reflect, I realized that my negative thoughts were compounding, and I started to feel as if I was losing my internal locus of control. I found myself scheming how to reduce my physician workload to spend the time I wanted to with my kids. There were times I wondered if I wanted to keep practicing medicine at all in the current system. Intellectually, I knew leaving medicine completely was not the solution because I truly love caring for patients, but I was becoming disenchanted with the productivity metrics and the extra administrative tasks replacing my time with patients. Fortunately, the concepts of lifestyle medicine resonated with my personal values and purpose for choosing a career in medicine, and I was able to reinvigorate my medical practice by changing the focus to health promotion, wellness, and disease reversal with my patients during their visits.

I became more consistent with my mindfulness practice and started to see its immense benefits. Up to this point, I had read several books on meditation and completed short workshops and yoga classes. However, it was after the intentional incorporation of meditation into my daily life that I started to see its positive effects. Mindfulness is the relationship between the mind and body, and it helps create awareness and space between the stimulus and the response. Rather than acting on default or reacting, I was more cognizant of how I wanted to respond to situations. By engaging in meditation and journaling, I could reflect and understand where I was causing my own unnecessary suffering. By meditating, I was alone with my thoughts. I could observe them without judgment or needing to change them. I noticed some of my habitual thoughts were perpetuating my burnout. Examples of unhelpful thoughts that kept me stuck were, "This isn't how it should be done. I don't have enough time with patients. Why do I have to do this administrative task?" I started to reframe the tasks and situations that were causing me the most distress—charting, in-basket management, short visits, and patient panel size, and I began to think of solutions or modifications where I had control within the broken medical system.

Another area where I deepened my mindfulness practice was taking time to be fully present with my young kids. It started with being forced to sit, relax, and nurse my babies. These periods of quiet relaxation, sometimes, allowed complete engagement with the present moment, and other times, necessary mind wandering and creativity. I also started to focus on small moments to completely immerse myself in their joy and contentment and be in awe of their learning and development.

As part of my time management planning, I started to carve out time to do activities I enjoyed. One such activity was indulging in my natural curiosity and reading books for pleasure. At first, it felt unnatural, and I worried I was not being productive, but paradoxically I started to be more focused and productive at work. I started by buying a Kindle but found it difficult to make the time for reading, so I adapted by listening to audiobooks or book summaries on my commute to work instead. This welcome distraction gave me another perspective to further evaluate my view of the world.

I made a consistent effort to journal, specifically focused on gratitude and celebrating accomplishments. I started small by writing down three things for which I was grateful or that I wanted to remember from that day. There is scientific evidence that we can train ourselves to focus on the positive and be more satisfied with life by engaging in a regular gratitude practice. It can be easy to find and focus on the negative in life. After all, our survival mechanism tells us to watch out for threats to keep us safe. However, our bodies often react with the same fight or flight response to the daily stressors of modern life that they would to a predator. Thankfully, we can recognize this in ourselves and intentionally activate our parasympathetic nervous system. For me, I was able to achieve this best with breathing, journaling, mindfulness, and gratitude.

I am grateful for having studied Lifestyle Medicine and intentionally applying its lessons to my personal and professional life, especially that of stress management. Lifestyle Medicine has been the antidote to my clinical burnout, allowing me to return to my purpose of caring for patients. Above all, the most meaningful lesson for me, and the one I hope to share with other healthcare providers, is that we cannot continue to promote self-sacrifice in our medical culture. Instead, by recognizing that we are our most important patient, and caring for our own well-being, will allow us to continually provide the quality care we strive to give.

This chapter is dedicated to all my compassionate, intelligent physician colleagues! It's such an honor to be part of a profession that can accompany patients through suffering and other times, contribute to medical miracles.

Thank you to my husband for all your love and support through it all and to my beautiful children, who are my everything. Thank you for providing my life with pure joy and reminding me how to stay present.

About Dr. Trisha Schimek, MD, MSPH, DipABLM

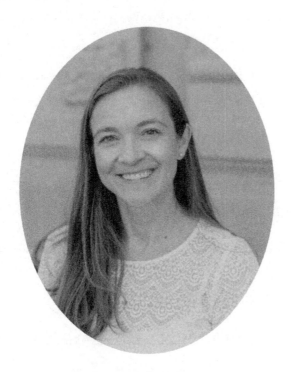

Dr. Trisha Schimek is board certified in Family Medicine and Lifestyle Medicine. She has dedicated her early medical career to working in under-resourced settings domestically and globally. She currently works in a California county health system as a primary care physician and faculty in a Family Medicine residency. She has a passion for helping her patients prevent and reverse chronic disease and loves celebrating her patient's success and motivating them through tough times. Beyond Lifestyle Medicine, she has expertise in comprehensive maternal and child health, reproductive justice, clinical procedures, medical education, provider well-being, and transgender health.

Professionally she did her undergraduate studies and master's of public health at Tulane University. She studied medicine at Jefferson Medical College and completed her Family Medicine residency at the University of Wisconsin, Madison. She is fellowship trained in global health and worked with the Indian Health Service and Partners in Health, Mexico while completing the UCSF Health Equity and Leadership (HEAL) Global Health Fellowship. She continues to mentor health professionals through this program.

Her interests outside of medicine include spending time with her husband and two young kids, traveling and exploring new places, searching for and creating nutritious recipes, reading, and anything that will take her outdoors: triathlons, hiking, biking, and camping.

Instagram: https://www.instagram.com/healthyfamilydoctor/

Website: https://healthyfamilydoctor.org/

LinkedIn: https://www.linkedin.com/in/trisha-schimek-md-mph-dipablm-42951544/

Watch an interview with the co-author:

Co-Author spotlight
DR. TRISHA SCHIMEK

Scan Me

26

The Journey Back to Myself

Wendy Schofer, MD, FAAP, DipABLM, TIPC, CHWC

"Health is an investment that we get to make in ourselves every day."

— Wendy Schofer, MD

T he language of medicine is pretty clear: eat this, move like this, take this, avoid that, and you'll be healthy. The language is laden with rules and is as clear as mud.

For years, though, I sought the elusive answers. They were "out there," far away from the location and culture where I grew up.

I was raised in suburban Pennsylvania Dutch Country. If you aren't familiar, God placed people in this beautiful area of southeastern PA to create the finest cured meats, cheeses, pies, casseroles, and baked goods. I loved sweet bologna and Lebanon bologna, Muenster cheese, and shoofly pie. Funnel cake was at all of the community events and considered a food group during festivals.

I went to college not far from my hometown and started learning that there were different ways to eat and move. Mostly I learned to avoid cheese and peanut butter as I learned that "all fats were bad," which vilified about 90% of the food I had eaten in childhood. I played sports as a child to be with my friends, not because I was particularly adept at any of them (I can count more teams I was cut from than ones I was included on).

In college, I found that my love of biology and genetics was not, in fact, lining me up to do forensic work because I found that the laboratory was a lonely place for me. Instead, I thrived connecting with people while I volunteered in the local emergency room. I decided to take my love of biology and genetics to medical school.

In medical school, I learned all "the rules" of what it meant to be healthy and what happened when you didn't follow those rules: you developed "disease." And I learned how to treat these diseases. I heard about the dangers of the diet I had grown up on and thanked my academic interests for getting me out of Pennsylvania Dutch Country.

Shortly thereafter, I started my active duty time in the Navy. I learned that I had to "run for my country" twice each year in the physical readiness test (PRT), and I started feeling pressure to make sure I would be able to weigh in "within standards" and be able to perform adequately on the PRT.

Meanwhile, I was rushed and harried. I had a young family, no time to myself, and barely any time with them. I grew anxious and depressed, yet I didn't even have the time to seek help. I was too busy following all the rules of what it meant to be a good doctor, wife, and mother. Over time, I learned that I had experienced burnout (several times) without having the words for it at the time.

I was living off of Pepsi One and as many peanut M&Ms as I could fit into the pockets of my white coat as I would head off to round on the wards for what seemed like a marathon. I ran because I had to. After all, my country and fear of the consequences of my Pennsylvania Dutch heritage depended on me running.

I was miserable.

I hit rock bottom at a time after I transferred with my family, yet again, to a new state. I found myself joyfully underemployed but also disconnected from my community.

I started exploring cooking more at home with my newfound time. I was stunned while walking by some CrossFit workouts and asked if that could be for me. I surprisingly found that I could enjoy movement, strength, and progress. (I also discovered that my grandfather had been a champion weightlifter: strength was in the family!) I explored yoga initially to recover from (yet another) running injury and found that I could learn to sit with myself, not having to move to prove anything. And I found sleep and connection within my community.

Shortly thereafter, I discovered Lifestyle Medicine (LM). Honest to goodness, I thought, "This is a thing?! This is what I've been doing!"

I was completely intrigued that there were others who were embracing movement, food, stress relief, and the beauty of connection to other humans. It was as if finding LM gave me permission to embrace what I had been finding actually worked for me over time.

Sleep. I need more sleep than the average person (9 hours on a regular basis). I was chronically sleep-deprived in training and my early career. No wonder it felt like the wheels were always about to come off. Sleep is now the default first answer when I notice things going sideways. Whenever I notice stress is more pronounced, I start craving atypical foods, and my emotions are amplified. I have learned to compassionately notice this happening and create a space for rest. In truth, rest is more than sleep. It is the fuel, the pacing, and the compassion that helps me see my truest humanity. I am not a machine. I am not waiting until I'm dead to rest or sleep, and sleep is not optional. Sleep comes first.

Food. Real food. The primacy of time and rushing had always seemed to get in the way of planning for real food to nourish my body and my family. We weren't eating a ton of junk, but convenience was key. As I learned more about nutrition and its impact on a multitude of factors (including academics, focus, and mental health), the more time I wanted to invest in creating nourishing meals for my entire family. Over time, I found that I was sampling one form of eating restriction, then another, in trying to find the "right diet." It didn't work. What I did find was that while I was trying to avoid my children developing restricted eating patterns, I actually had my own. Today, my husband calls me the "95% vegetarian." I tell him to stop doing the math about what I eat. LM has taught me so much about listening to what my body needs, more so than needing to follow a strict dietary pattern. My body loves a variety of foods—just not meat.

Movement. Moving out of fear of disease or of "not making the cut" on a military physical readiness test is bananas. Moving out of fear is exactly what we do when we are stressed in classic stress-cycle demonstrations. But that is not the only way to move our bodies. I learned that I can move out of joy and create more joy for myself while moving. Our bodies need movement to function properly, and I found that I need movement as a daily part of my mental health support. This was recognized out of love, not out of fear or a mandate to move a certain way. How refreshing!

Movement for joy and mental health is something that I have actively found myself sharing with others. There is a cultural assumption that movement is exercise and mandated. I discovered that does not have to be the truth, and actively share with my children how I feel during and after movement. I ask them what they are experiencing to invite viewing movement as a way to explore what their bodies are capable of and to get to learn more about their bodies.

Connection. Connection is my jam. I realized that I had never taken a single course in psychology through all of my training in college and medicine. Yes, I had studied developmental pediatrics, psychiatry, and a whole lot of psychopharmacology. I could "fix" what was broken. But I had never had the opportunity to understand what our brains do: we are wired for connection. I dove into positive psychology, the psychology of change, and trauma. All of these areas are founded in the human need for connection, which was missing for so much of my own training and early career. Connection is such a powerful motivator for me. It is truly the emotion that drives the vast majority of my actions, and it helps me connect with other parents in my clinical practice as well as my coaching practice. Connection is human healing.

Stress management. At the heart of all of our modern diseases is stress. Stress is external in the form of obligations and expectations, and circumstances beyond our control. And yet, there is such a wealth of internal stress that can only be addressed when we give ourselves the loving opportunity to become aware of it, examine it, question it, and consider alternative approaches. Viktor Frankl is quoted about finding the space between stimulus and response being our opportunity to choose, grow, and be free. Well, I choose to find the space between stressors and the assumption that I will be stressed about them. Our modern society has stressors that we can't just run away from, like the saber-tooth tiger stressor that our ancestors experienced. Our stressors follow us by taking space between our ears: to-do lists, weight fears, obligations, and time management. The combination of addressing our own perceptions of the importance of those stressors, as well as the institutional and cultural changes that are needed to address the external circumstances, still starts with recognizing the power that we have as individuals to address our own stress. Keep in mind that I am a registered yoga instructor, and it is only now that I mention yoga and meditation. They are amazing methodologies, and yet just a part of the toolkit we can mobilize for personal stress management. Heck, it took me over 10 years of practicing yoga to find it as a stress-management option, as I was initially using it for enjoyable movement. And that is okay!

Avoidance of substance. We all want to belong, and when we are in pain, we look to numb the discomfort. The substance can be tobacco, plants, pharmaceuticals, alcohol, or food. The LM pillar of avoiding substances reminds me to be mindful if I am consuming to enjoy it or to numb discomfort.

My burnout story and my introduction to LM brought me to the most important thing, myself. I realized that I wasn't the problem, and I sure wasn't broken. I was just living according to someone else's rules, and *they didn't fit me*. I wasn't living according to what was nourishing to my body and soul. This journey along which I encountered LM has offered me the opportunity to grant myself permission to see what was right in my life and what I wanted more of. I also was able to unlearn the concept of health that was taught to me in medical school. Health isn't the absence of disease. It isn't a particular weight, and it's not defined by biomarkers or by anyone else, for that matter. Health is personal, and it is an investment that you get to make each and every day.

These are the tenets by which I live my life now:

– Find what is going well

– Ask what I want more of

– Ask how am I investing in myself each and every day

– Give myself permission to be unapologetically me

– Never having to be somewhere else to experience what is most important to me

That looks like being connected to myself and my family, sleeping nine hours each and every night, eating a (95% according to my husband) whole food plant-based diet, moving when I want and how I want, working (and loving!) clinical medicine on my terms, and building a sustainable business that nourishes me. My life, my lifestyle, my health. This is the model of healthcare that I share with my family, patients, clients, and community. We all can.

This chapter is dedicated to the exhausted pediatric resident Dr. Schofer who had the critical voices turned up way too loud. Your strength is in your vulnerability. The journey will always be to be more you, Love. You can give yourself permission to rest. And when you're ready, consider weightlifting. Lifting, dropping, and cussing help you uncover a new type of strength. Much love -W

About Dr. Wendy Schofer, MD, FAAP, DipABLM, TIPC, CHWC

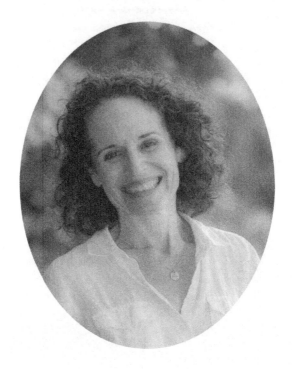

Dr. Wendy Schofer is a holistic pediatrician and lifestyle medicine physician and certified life & body image coach for families. As the founder of Family in Focus, she specializes in helping parents struggling with their children's weight to create better lifelong relationships with food, body, and family by using cognitive behavioral coaching tools, and trauma-informed and feminist methodologies. She connects with parents through humor and stories of real-life struggles and tools for creating health at home on her podcast, *Family in Focus with Wendy Schofer, MD.*

- Board Certified Pediatrician

- Board Certified Lifestyle Physician

- Certified Life & Weight Coach (The Life Coach School)

- Certified Health & Wellness Coach (Wellcoaches)

- Certified Neuro-Linguistic Programming Coach (Symbiosis)

- Certified Trauma-Informed Professional Coach (Lodestar)

- Advanced Certification in Feminist Coaching (in progress—because we are all works in progress)

- Registered Yoga Teacher (RYT-200)

- CrossFit Level 1 Trainer

- Twenty years of making health fun and easy

Website: https://www.wendyschofermd.com/

Instagram: www.instagram.com/wendyschofermd

LinkedIn: https://www.linkedin.com/in/wendy-schofer-md-735b948

Podcast: https://podcasts.apple.com/us/podcast/family-in-focus-with -wendy-schofer-md/id1571510508

Watch an interview with the co-author:

Co-Author spotlight
DR. WENDY SCHOFER

Scan Me

27

FINDING MY IKIGAI: LIFESTYLE MEDICINE

Mythri Shankar, MBBS, MD (USA), DipIBLM, AFMCP

"God, grant me the serenity to accept the things I cannot change, courage to change the things I can, and wisdom to know the difference."

— Reinhold Niebuhr

It was in Rome when I was giving a talk at the World Congress of Osteoporosis that I learned two things—that Italian gelato is every bit as delicious as it's claimed to be and those gladiators (the big tall, muscular guys who could fight a lion with their bare hands at the Colosseum) were vegetarian.

Food has always been at the center of good health. Plant-based foods are sufficient. I wasn't surprised by this fact since I already knew this from my own experience of being a vegetarian my entire life.

My Background

I am a physician who has been practicing for well over 25 years. I have been impressed by legendary cardiologists like Dr. Dean Ornish and Dr.

K. Lance Gould, pioneers in cardiac health and imaging (PET-CT) at the University of Texas, USA. I was the first to apply for a license in California to use the positron PET-CT scanner in a private practice outpatient setting after purchasing a used cardiac PET-CT scanner.

But, when I returned to India in 2005, I realized that I was armed with knowledge that could not be applied here—because only around ten hospitals in the whole country had the basic facility for PET-CT (cancer imaging), let alone cardiac PET-CT. What caught me by surprise was the lack of awareness and the absence of basic medical equipment for osteoporosis, which is an easily preventable disease, also rampantly underdiagnosed and poorly understood by patients and doctors alike. Eventually, I turned my attention from the heart to osteoporosis, which led to that moment in Rome, where I saw food in a new light.

My Personal History

After returning to India, I was diagnosed with type 2 diabetes after having gestational diabetes in the past. My mother has been a diabetic for over 30 years. My mother likely also had gestational diabetes, but it was not something routinely checked in pregnancy during that time. I was prescribed metformin, which has numerous side effects that will make you think of not giving this medicine to anyone: heartburn, stomach pain, nausea, vomiting, bloating, gas, diarrhea, constipation, weight loss, and headache. Additionally, it leaves an unpleasant metallic taste in the mouth. The only positive of metformin that held appeal was weight loss. "But was it worth all this suffering?" I asked myself.

I wondered if I could reverse my diabetes without medication by turning to food. And thus began my adventure with food, the diseases it causes, and other lifestyle-related parameters.

In clinical practice, there were constant questions from my patients about why they were developing diseases without any risk factors. And then I had some questions myself — why did I develop diabetes? I was over 45 years old. My BMI was normal. I've been a vegetarian all my life. Now, I was wondering if I really needed this drug called metformin. Once I started taking it, I'd probably have to take it my whole life, just like my mom. Just thinking of its side effects was enough to give me a bad taste in my mouth. Nothing about this medication sounded appealing except for the weight loss bit. It sounded like a vicious cycle. So, my search for medical literature on another cure for diabetes began again.

My Introduction to Reversing Disease

After browsing thousands of web pages, watching hundreds of videos by famous doctors who worked on plant-based food and on diabetes reversal programs, and reading 60 to 70 books (thanks to Kindle and Amazon's delivery, despite the lockdown), I was finally convinced. Yes, this can work. Every patient of mine needs to give this "reverse disease concept by lifestyle modifications" a try. But why didn't anyone tell me this before? Why weren't doctors emphasizing the lifestyle aspects which can bring about a reversal of disease? Why do doctors assume it is difficult for the patient to change? Or, is it easier for them to prescribe medicines rather than counsel change?

In modern society, it has almost become a norm to accept lifestyle-related diseases as a natural course of human aging. They are not. These are purely man-made and can be prevented and reversed simply by questioning the systems' paradigms and the beliefs they stand on. There is ample evidence now to support the belief that lifestyle changes can reduce disease burden. *You* hold the key to unlocking the answer to the million-dollar question of your life's "quantity" and "quality": how long and how well you will live. All you need to do is put some effort into turning the key in the right direction.

Integrating My Expertise

Being a Nuclear Medicine physician with 25 years of clinical practice, I am trained to look at functional imaging and the physiological parameters of organs at a cellular level using unique radioisotopes. This allows doctors to see more than what usually meets the eye (beyond the anatomy) in a physical exam or radiological imaging (like X-ray, ultrasound, or CT scan). So, my field is patient-centric and rarely industry-driven. For instance, Cardiac Stress Myocardial Perfusion Imaging shows if heart bypass surgery or a stent is really needed or if it can be managed medically in a non-invasive way (without surgery). Similarly, in DEXA scans, we look at hidden or visceral fat. Similarly, PET-CT scans are done using special radioisotopes like FDG, a glucose analog that mimics glucose and goes wherever glucose goes, particularly in high concentrations to cancer cells as tumor cells feed on glucose and grow faster. These scans show the extent and depth of the spread of cancer. I used this knowledge of bodily functions to work on my diabetes. And I have been able to reverse my diabetes successfully (my beginning HbA1c was 7.8, now down to HbA1c < 6), mainly with lifestyle modifications and no medications.

Lifestyle Diseases

The ultimate realization dawned on me: the many typical reasons most of our loved ones die early can all be prevented with lifestyle changes. When looking at the numbers, statistics can make it seem hopeless. Heart disease is the #1 killer of patients over 50 years of age; 62% of the cancer is already in Stage 3 or 4, and a majority of diabetics are overweight or obese. Bones break because they weren't taken care of with proper nutrition. Knee pain and joint pain actually arise because of neglect from wear and tear. The common denominator to all these conditions I had been working on all my life in my specialty of Nuclear Medicine—heart disease, osteoporosis, cancer, diabetes, autoimmune diseases like thyroiditis, or the hormonal influences on endocrine organs (be it the thyroid or the pancreas, or renal complications due to diabetes), neurological problems like Parkinson's or Alzheimer's—is *one's lifestyle: the way you live your life, how you treat your body, which houses your mind, soul, and well-being*. All of these diseases are preventable and reversible. But only if we make the right choices, keeping ourselves in mind.

Giving Back to Yourself

I see everyone fret about minor things on the outside. The most important "things" in life are not things at all. We give more importance to the type of gas or petrol we put into our cars than the food we put into our bodies. We pay more attention to the texture of the upholstery on our sofas than to the layers coating the blood vessels on the inside. We give more importance to the deposits made into our bank accounts rather than the fat accumulating within our bodies. These diseases are a "normal" response to an "abnormal" way of living. It's our lifestyle that is the culprit here. The body always does what it is supposed to do. It is programmed to do the best it can with what it is given and never gives up on you. Even inflammation is a protective body response. But inflammation works against the body too. It is caused by what you put inside the body and cannot be stopped by the body alone. Symptoms are the body's way of calling for help. Modern medicine has much to understand about the human body. And medication is only putting a Band-Aid on the problem without addressing the real issue. Your body is not your enemy; it's your friend. Don't restrict it. Nourish it and lovingly take care of it.

Taking Care of Myself

My interest in yoga started when I was in my first year at medical school. Yoga was a treatment option to control my allergies and sinusitis. Jal Neti Yoga (Kriya) seemed to help. It was taught meticulously at Vivekananda Yoga Kendra in Bangalore. During my third year at the ENT posting at Wenlock Hospital in Mangalore, I realized that Jasl Neti yoga is nothing but an anterior nasal wash, a physical detox process, which, when done repeatedly, desensitizes the nasal mucosa and helps build the body's resistance.

Combined Experience

I am trained and licensed to practice medicine, and I am a citizen of the USA and India. My experience over 25 years combines the best of both worlds: learnings from the latest technological advances by the pioneers in the Western world and certain late realizations about Eastern philosophies. The built-in ideology which every Indian is born with is our integrated and interdependent relationship with nature in a predominantly vegetarian country, home to yoga and spirituality. New discoveries only validate our traditional way of living again and again. India's history could provide answers to modern world issues such as climate change, animal rights, and morality and ethics, as we now see, based on emerging evidence in science that is validating our age-old practices.

Current medicine is not as effective for cures and economic costs as it is meant to be. With lifestyle medicine, we can change this and bring certain matters to the forefront, reducing healthcare costs. Like Dr. Dennis Bukett said, "If people are constantly falling off the cliff, we need to build fences around those cliffs, not place ambulances under them." Doctors don't get paid for lifestyle counseling or diet coaching. We are trained to *treat* disease, not so much to *prevent* it. Health needs to be reformed when the rubber meets the road. Lifestyle Medicine is the answer.

The paradigm of "reversing disease" is not in medical textbooks or current medical practice. Doctors are trained in Anatomy, Physiology, Biochemistry, Microbiology, Pathology, Pharmacology, Forensic Medicine, Dentistry, Surgery, Medicine Obstetrics, and Gynecology. A medical internship also mainly focuses on clinical aspects of the same subjects. We have not been taught nutrition, disease reversal, or to promote wellness until now. We treat and manage disease. Or refer the patient to a dietician or a nutritionist.

We need an integrated system in our fast-paced modern era. Doctors are not trained to learn and practice the health influencers like diet, physical activity, sleep hygiene, stress management, positive psychology, and risky substance abuse, which form an integrated healing process for the human body. Nor do they have the time for this. The amount of nutrition education in medical schools remains inadequate.

Salutogenesis versus Pathogenesis

When we are taught prevention, it is in the context of community medicine with a focus on infectious diseases. "Pathogenesis" is all about the pathogen and the birth of disease. It has been explained well in all medical textbooks, over and over again. But "Salutogenesis" is quite the opposite. It focuses on well-being, health, stress, and coping. This concept was initially developed while studying the survivors of the Holocaust. At first, it was hard to wrap my head around these new concepts, which are sustainable and lifesaving. There are higher principles involved here, going beyond just being vegan and not waiting for an extreme medical trigger to change our health. Nutrition, movement, and connectedness to people and the environment can build our body's resilience and resistance to disease. There is no judgment in any shape or form here. Yes, it is possible to un-script or re-script your body's prescription for health.

Whether you relate to Plato's microcosm-macrocosm analogy or the Indian *Aham Brahmasmi* philosophy, there should be humility in acknowledging the fact that what we know (limited intelligence) is significantly less than what we don't (infinite ignorance). Rahul Dravid and Einstein are great exemplars of humility and modesty. Having an open mindset toward the other accepted modalities of Integrated Medicine: Ayurveda, acupuncture, yoga, movement therapy (like Tai Chi), massage therapy, biofeedback, etc., can help us heal. These evidence-based and strong approaches complement modern medicine, not detract from it.

Scientific Measures of Health

We can now measure several vital biochemicals, which helps us analyze functional deficiencies at the cellular level. Numbers make it simpler for us to understand and provide evidence to the questions our cerebral mind often seeks. Functional tests are now available. For example, one can have a panel of tests for inflammatory cardiac markers due to stress, stool analysis, and breath tests for gut health, telomere testing for aging or oxidative stress-free radicals. We can also measure nutritional parameters in our body, such as vitamins, minerals (Calcium, Magnesium, Manganese, Zinc, Copper), amino acids (Asparagine, Glutamine, Serine), fatty acids (Oleic Acid), antioxidants (Alpha Lipoic Acid, Coenzyme Q10, Cysteine, Glutathione, Selenium, Vitamin E), carbohydrate metabolism (Chromium, Fructose Sensitivity, Glucose-Insulin Metabolism), metabolites (Choline, Inositol, Carnitine), Total Antioxidant Function, and Immune Response Score. A cardiac panel, including Lipoprotein Fractionation, Lipoprotein Particle Numbers, Total Cholesterol, Total LDL Particles, Total HDL Particles, Triglycerides, Lipoprotein (a), hs-CRP, Homocysteine, Apolipoprotein A-1, Apolipoprotein B, and insulin can give meaningful information.

Genetic testing, like telomere testing, predicts cellular death, which causes the body to age, thus making telomeres novel biomarkers of biological age. Telomere shortening, when expedited, contributes to cardiovascular disease, dementia, stroke, and cancer. The MTHFR test measures methylation, which is involved in many biological pathways and can detect impaired detoxification, cardiovascular disease, neurological problems, and weakened immune functioning in general. Telomeres are an integrative index of many lifetime influences — the restorative ones like good fitness and sleep and malignant ones like toxic stress, poor nutrition, and other adversities. Thus, it has been suggested that telomere length may be the Holy Grail for cumulative welfare, to be used as a summative measure of our life experiences.

While these tests are valuable, we need a broader approach. Having a good quality of life and longevity are inseparable and intricately intertwined. Lifestyle can be modified only by taking ownership of your life. Focus on yourself in a deep, holistic sense, and not just on numbers like weight, blood sugar, or cholesterol level. As a doctor, I like to treat and heal patients, not just improve the chart. My principle is: Follow Saraswati (an abstract symbol of knowledge and wisdom), and Lakshmi (a symbol of financial wealth) will automatically follow. Health is wealth, and both are counted in numbers. And a prayer to Durga (protector of right and destroyer of all things wrong). Pray that she gives you the courage to change what you can, the serenity to accept the things you cannot change, and the wisdom to see the difference.

Our Current State of Health

It is mind-boggling to see the obesity epidemic and how food manufacturing companies subconsciously manipulate our eating habits and food choices. We are now dealing with the social dynamics of an unhealthy food culture. Obesity is linked to 40% of the 13 major cancers, including brain, breast, thyroid, stomach, liver, pancreas, kidney, ovaries, uterus, and colon cancers. Obesity accounts for 80–85% of the risk of developing type 2 diabetes and is among the leading causes of elevated cardiovascular disease (CVD) mortality and morbidity. Being overweight by just 20 pounds increases the risk of stroke by 24% and the risk of developing depression by 55 %.

Lifestyle disease numbers are growing fast. They are called lifestyle diseases because they are man-made and self-imposed. The good news is about 50–60% of them can be managed without medication. Some lifestyle diseases can be avoided altogether if these changes are adopted early.

Lifestyle medicine (LM) is based on six pillars: nutrition, physical activity, stress, sleep, substance abuse, and positive psychology/social connection. LM is a newly added specialty, although it may appear as old wine in a new bottle to some. LM focuses on preventive aspects and self-care based on research. LM treats the root cause of disease by modifying lifestyle factors such as nutrition, physical inactivity, chronic stress, poor sleep, and bad habits (smoking, alcohol consumption, etc.). As a primary modality, LM is delivered by doctors who are trained and tested in it. The sum total of my life's experiences (both personal and professional) inspired me to officially pursue this specialty and become board-certified internationally, adding value to my existing credentials and war chest to treat patients.

Success Stories

It has been amazing to learn how patients have reversed lifestyle diseases like diabetes, hypertension, obesity, arthritis, etc., and are now living comfortably without medication. Some cases are borderline, but they can still avoid medication through strict and vigilant lifestyle modifications. A diet consisting predominantly of fruits, vegetables, legumes, nuts, seeds, and plant protein, central to a whole food plant-based (WFPB) diet, can prevent heart disease. Restricting saturated fat and dietary cholesterol intake and increasing the intake of fiber-rich foods can help control one's lipid profile better. Eating a low sodium-high potassium diet along with a WFPB diet can help prevent and treat hypertension. Body weight and healthy calorie restriction are vital for preventing diabetes, but as my personal history shows, they are not enough. LM and a WFPB were necessary.

Serendipity

Life has given me a chance to pursue my current passion for living healthily and naturally. My goal now is to get people off unnecessary medication and help them understand the profound effect food, self-esteem, sex, survival, status, spirituality, function, family, and relationships can have on the golden years of life. I have gotten to explore the analogies between the scientific evidence over multiple concepts—micro-macro chasms, Zeitgerbers, circadian rhythm, fight or flight/rest and digest cycles, salutogenesis, dysbiosis, gut microbiota, epigenetics, adaptogens, parasympathetic nervous system, the vagus nerve, the DOPA trap, the healing powers of integrated medicine and spirituality, etc.—and now I know how to use all this knowledge of organ intelligence and biohack neuroplasticity to move our bodies to healthier lifescapes with emotional intelligence without succumbing to the seductive influence of SOS (sugar, oil, salt).

Lifestyle Medicine has a place in modern medicine and, in fact, should be a priority. Recent advances in technology are supposed to make life better but, unfortunately, the detrimental effects that technology has on one's health have actually made life worse. Despite research correlating the effects of air pollution, soil pollution, and water pollution on human health, the numbers in the world's bank balance are becoming more important than the numbers on the blood report. Corruption and pollution are becoming the norm instead of being exceptions. The havoc that the media has created on our health is indisputable. The biology of stress on the human body is evident. Do yourself a favor: stop the constant worry about earning more, acquiring more, competing for more, stressing over meaningless things, etc. Remember, the most important things in life aren't things at all!

Lifestyle Medicine is my IKIGAI

The COVID-19 pandemic-induced lockdown forced us to slow down, rethink, reprioritize, and stop overdoing certain things and instead focus on the meaning and purpose of whatever we do. It has given me a chance to reflect upon life, find a way to give back to the community, grow, bond, and share. Perhaps it is the plant-generated oxygen's positive effect on my endorphins, but I can nourish myself better. I can experience joy, patience, and humility. The perfectionist in me has been a silent witness to how lifestyle causes disease. Modern medicine sometimes overlooks the cause of the illnesses and the downward spirals they cause. Our focus shouldn't be only on compliance and complacence with corporate mandates but also on community service elements. I have always placed paramount importance on education and the continuous pursuit of excellence as the highest virtue. I have always followed my passion with an unerring and innate sense of direction, beginning with a desire to practice evidence-based medicine both in the diagnostic and therapeutic arena of modern medicine. The COVID-19 pandemic lockdown and my diagnosis of diabetes introduced me to Lifestyle Medicine—My IKIGAI, my newfound "motivating force." Interacting with the LM community of doctors—I am so glad to have finally found my tribe and share how to thrive.

This chapter is dedicated to my fellow physicians who work tirelessly to serve their patients. More power to them in finding their own meaning and purpose in their respective professions - just like I found mine (Ikigai).

About Dr. Mythri Shankar, MBBS, MD(USA), DipIBLM, AFM-CP

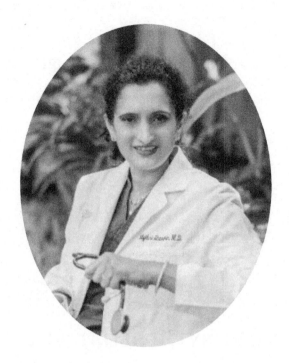

- Board Certified Lifestyle Medicine Physician

- Specialized in Nuclear Medicine: Nuclear Cardiology, Nuclear Oncology, Theranostics, Radioisotope Therapies, and Osteoporosis

- Author

- TEDx Speaker

- Award-winning organic gardener

- Health Activist

- Environmentalist

- Ethical Vegan

- Culinary Medicine Enthusiast

- Author, <u>Ease: How to Lose Weight, Heal, Prevent and Reverse Disease</u>

Instagram: <u>https://www.instagram.com/thegreenfoundationindia</u>

LinkedIn: <u>https://www.linkedin.com/in/drmythrishankar/</u>

TEDx talk link: <u>https://youtu.be/H57NYSlItb8</u>

Facebook: <u>https://www.facebook.com/tgfi.greenhub.7</u>

<u>Watch an interview with the co-author:</u>

Co-Author spotlight
DR. MYTHRI SHANKAR

Scan Me

28

Empowered: A Physician's Journey from Parental Health to Personal Health

Saba Sharif, MD, FAAAI, DipABLM

"Don't let your learning lead to knowledge. Let your learning lead to action."

— Jim Rohn

"Your father is having chest pain, and we are going to the ER." A few hours later, there was another update. "The doctors say he needs heart bypass surgery."

I was in California during my fellowship training when my mom called from New York and relayed these alarming messages a few hours apart. My father had felt severe burning in his chest after shoveling snow. The hospital doctors told him that cholesterol deposits narrowed his coronary arteries (blood vessels to the heart). Our entire family was stunned. My father had always been a thin, active nonsmoker and did not have high-risk factors for heart disease such as high blood pressure, high cholesterol, or diabetes. I wanted to be there with him, as a concerned daughter, to offer moral support and as a physician to speak to his doctors. But I was 3,000 miles away, feeling helpless, holding my breath and praying that he would be okay.

Soon after his surgery, he flew in to visit me and had chest pain again while moving his luggage, so we took him to the local emergency room (ER). His bypassed grafts had failed, his heart was leaking enzymes from the stress of the exertion, and his original arteries needed to be opened immediately! The cardiologist opened his blocked arteries by placing metal stents throughout them. I was relieved, until we asked what would happen if he had this type of chest pain again. The response was, 'nothing else can be done,' besides medications. The doctor shared that this would be the last procedure that could be done for my dad's heart since the blood vessels needed for the bypass had already been used and failed. Since then, whenever my dad complained of chest tightness with fast or uphill walking, the doctors proposed medications alone to help his symptoms. Hearing 'nothing else can be done' to reduce the risk of death weighed on our family like a dark gray cloud. Eventually, I moved to the east coast to be closer to him, knowing I was only a few hours away in case he had heart issues again.

A decade later, I received a frantic call—this time from my father. "Your mother isn't waking up. Should I call 911?!" In disbelief, I exclaimed, "What do you mean?!" I had just spoken to her the night before. He switched the call to FaceTime so I could see her on video; I will never forget witnessing my mom unresponsive and the feelings that came with it. It felt like a nightmare, but it was also a crisis that I needed to fix. The patient was my mom. Under surreal circumstances, I somehow guided my dad through the next steps. The paramedics arrived and took her to the ER. Soon after, the doctor called to inform me that my mother had suffered a severe brain injury. Only when I took a back seat, literally and figuratively, on the hours-long car ride to the ER did I allow myself to cry and my feelings to flow. It was devastating to see my mother responding with only eye and head movements when she was the most lively and cheerful person I had known.

Desperate to get the matriarch of our family back, I searched the literature for similar cases and spoke to specialists. My family and I were determined to give her the best chance of recovery. Thankfully, she got accepted into a neurorehabilitation program, and we were hopeful.

I was at my mother's bedside all day, half of every week, to do my part to stimulate her recovery and take care of her. For the next couple of years, I was stretched to my limit as I continued to work in my practice and serve as her healthcare proxy, and traveled 10 hours weekly between states. I would have gone to the ends of the earth for my devoted mother, just as she had always championed us.

Her physical therapists prescribed specific exercises to flex and extend her limbs to keep her joints mobile. We continued these exercises daily while talking to her, communicating our love and trying to encourage her. Through touch and movement, we expressed to her that we were committed to her every step of the way and readying her for when she could move on her own again. The exercises were intended to keep supple my mother's arms, which used to give me enthusiastic bear hugs, and her legs, which used to walk down the stairs, as she would be the first one to greet me. "Movement is life," one of her physical therapists declared. What a concise yet profound statement that captured her big picture.

Before this tragedy, my mother had always been on the move; she walked and worked with purpose and efficiency. She also always focused on gratitude and often reminded us of the verse of the Quran, "If you are grateful, I will certainly give you more" (Abraham 14:7). I was grateful to be able to move my limbs and hers. Active movement *is* life. *I could never take for granted my ability to move again.* Just to be able to move my arms and take steps with my legs were movements I started to be mindful of when walking. I reflected on the brain-to-muscle communication needed with each of my movements and had a newfound appreciation of those simple movements as gifts to take advantage of.

Unfortunately, my mom could no longer choose movement, and her flexibility diminished over time. It sunk in that she would no longer welcome us with her exuberant hugs or uplift us with her smile and laughter. My beloved mother eventually succumbed to complications of prolonged immobility. She passed away after touching so many in her lifetime with joy and service.

My caregiving for two years had taken a toll on me. I was stressed about my mother and had a sedentary lifestyle during that time, eating at the train station or hospital cafeteria. I had unprecedented weight gain, disrupted sleep, and high blood pressure during those years. I looked in the mirror and didn't recognize the person looking back at me. I could not fit into my clothes anymore. After my mother passed away in 2020, my mental and physical health was at an all-time low. I needed to prioritize myself and turn my health around.

Transitioning to My Own Health

One day, Canadian Fitness Instructor Specialist Amina Khan caught my attention online. I started to feel glimmers of joy listening to her cheer on her followers during her YouTube exercises. I was attracted to her infectious positive energy. I became motivated to do something for myself for the first time in years. I started doing her 5-minute workouts and reduced my portion sizes at dinner. After a month, I built on my momentum and began doing her extended 20-minute workouts and taking brisk walks outdoors. Getting movement and feeling the sun and wind was uplifting. It was better than staying indoors, sad from the loss of my mother. Exercise released positive hormones, also known as 'endorphin highs,' and became an empowering tool for my self-care. Changing my diet and exercise had positive results that gave me a sense of control over my well-being, in contrast to the helplessness I had felt over the slow loss of my mom. I also started following Amina Khan's nutrition content and reading her healthy eating tips. She shared the dangers of sugar, how it stimulates pleasure centers in our brains and is as addictive as cocaine. I accepted her challenge to eliminate added sugar entirely from my diet for seven days. What started as one week of abstinence from added sugar continued well beyond. Despite my reputable sweet tooth, I no longer had an appetite for something so harmful to my body.

I set my birthday as the target date to reach my weight goal, and it gave me something positive to focus on. The pounds kept shedding as I tallied my daily calories and tracked my daily weight. I lost twenty pounds over two and a half months! The intentional weight loss and clean living empowered me at a time when grief would have otherwise consumed me. I posted on social media about my success and inspired a few friends who asked me to join in whatever I was doing. This request led me to create "Mindfully Healthy," an accountability group of friends centered on our health goals.

Introduction to Lifestyle Medicine and Its Impact on My Health

While I was already becoming healthier, two of my physician friends mentioned studying for a new specialty called the Lifestyle Medicine (LM) boards. I learned that Lifestyle Medicine focuses on evidence-based approaches to prevent, treat, and reverse many chronic diseases. I was intrigued. Our traditional medical school and residency training focused on treating illness with medication, not on prevention or nutrition. I was reminded of my Internal Medicine (IM) residency training when I saw the same patients with diabetes or COPD (a type of lung disease) return to the hospital frequently with progressive disease and complications. These hospitalizations were due to failed treatments or non-adherence. Often, physicians did not have time for detailed lifestyle discussions and outsourced this to the nutritionist and social worker, so management was compartmentalized. The new specialty of Lifestyle Medicine offered hope that physicians could help patients by focusing just as much time, if not more, on lifestyle changes as on medications. This knowledge could help my dad with his heart disease, help me with my blood pressure and weight, and help the lives of the patients I touch. I decided to pursue it.

We formed an LM board review group of 10 physicians and studied together on Zoom three days weekly for months. We discussed the studies providing evidence for the six LM pillars. We learned about the Blue Zones Project—the five locations where people live the longest worldwide. These populations share nine characteristics: moving naturally (physical activity), having a sense of purpose, eating mainly a plant-based diet, eating until 80% full, relaxing, downshifting, putting family first, belonging to something greater, and finding the right tribe. Our study group explored practical ways to bring it all home.

> ### Did you know this about cholesterol and heart disease?
>
> - The top sources of cholesterol in the US diet are eggs 25%, chicken 12.5%, beef 11%, cheese 4.2%, and pork 3.9%.
> - "Atherosclerosis (buildup of plaque, that includes cholesterol, in arteries supplying blood to the heart) does not progress when low-density lipoprotein (LDL) cholesterol is less than 70 mg/dl" [1] and total cholesterol is less than 150 mg/dl" [2].
> - Coronary artery disease (hardening and narrowing of arteries supplying blood to the heart due to plaque buildup) is almost nonexistent in civilizations where diets are plant-based and low in fat. The diet in rural China compared to the diet in the United States had about half the fat, one-tenth of the meat intake, and three times the fiber intake; therefore, the average total cholesterol was only 127 mg/dl in rural China, but 203 mg/dl in the US [3].

After learning so much, I wanted to take stock of my health and have a baseline from which to improve. I finally visited my primary care doctor after a two-year delay due to caregiving. Lab results showed that my low-density lipoprotein (LDL) cholesterol, sometimes called 'bad' cholesterol, was on the high end of the normal range (up to 100 mg/dl LDL cholesterol is 'normal' according to most lab standards). Given my family history of severe heart disease, I wanted to make sure that I was not developing cholesterol deposits. I made it my personal goal to achieve cholesterol levels at which plaque buildup stops in the arteries supplying the heart, i.e., an LDL cholesterol of less than 70 mg/dl and total cholesterol of less than 150 mg/dl. I changed my diet to meet my cholesterol goals. I began to minimize processed foods, eliminate meat except fish, reduce eggs to once weekly, and limit fat-free dairy to nonfat Greek yogurt. Incorporating fish into my diet added healthy LDL-reducing anti-inflammatory omega-3 fatty acids. I reached my cholesterol targets in three months; my LDL cholesterol dropped 30 points, and my total cholesterol dropped 40 points! After already exercising and avoiding added sugar, screening for saturated fat led to another 10-pound weight loss. I reached my lowest weight, yet maintained a healthy body mass index (BMI). How empowering it was to know that when I set my mind to my health goals, I could achieve them with focus and commitment!

Did you know this about processed foods?

- Heavily processed foods often include unhealthy levels of fat, added sugar and salt, and low amounts of fiber that can lead to heart disease, high blood pressure, and diabetes.
- Most of the sugars consumed today are hidden in processed foods. For example, a single can of sugar-sweetened soda contains up to 40 grams (10 teaspoons) of free sugars. Also, one tablespoon of ketchup contains around 4 grams (around one teaspoon) of free sugar.
- The World Health Organization (WHO) recommends that people consume less than 5% (with a maximum of 10%) of total calories from free sugars daily. Five percent is equivalent to 6 teaspoons or 24 grams of added sugar per day. Free sugar refers to any added sugar, as well as sugars naturally present in honey, syrup, and fruit juices. In 2017—18, US adults' average sugar intake was 17 teaspoons of added sugar daily.
- WHO has determined that processed meats, such as ham, bacon, and salami, cause cancer, specifically increasing the risk of colon, stomach, pancreatic and prostate cancer. WHO also determined that red meat, such as beef, lamb, goat, and pork, probably cause colorectal cancer.

Cooking from scratch to avoid processed foods became a new adventure. Being in the kitchen used to feel like a chore, but now I like the challenge of cooking healthy dishes that taste delicious. My favorite homemade and vegetarian breakfast dishes to prepare and eat are oat pancakes with freshly made date and mango syrups, avocado toast, carrot and sweet potato lentils, and vegetable egg white omelets. These breakfasts have fueled my mornings and kept me light on my feet.

Did you know this about physical activity?

- A study following people over 45 years of age found that 6.9% of all causes of death were related to sitting time [4].
- Standing for two hours a day is associated with a 10% reduction in death from all causes [5].
- Exercise is equivalent to medications as secondary prevention of coronary artery disease and prediabetes. Benefits in cardiovascular disease reduction occur with 15 minutes per day or 90 minutes per week of moderate-intensity exercise [6].
- All-cause mortality (death) is reduced with 150 minutes of moderate-intensity or 75 minutes of vigorous activity per week [7].
- The CDC helps define moderate-intensity activity with the talk test; you can talk but not sing during the activity.

I am walking the walk, both literally and figuratively. The risk of dying prematurely declines as people become more physically active. Inspired by LM physician Dr. Michael Greger, who routinely gives talks while walking on his treadmill, I even have a desk treadmill now to keep me moving at my home desk. Every week, I aim to meet the national recommendation of 150 minutes of moderate-intensity exercise.

Aside from healthy eating and increasing physical activity, positive social connectedness and stress management are two more pillars of LM that have been important to my well-being. I connected socially through virtual groups during the pandemic. I created an online support group to process grief with other physicians like myself who have lost a parent. I developed growth-oriented connections through a social-emotional intelligence program at the Wright Foundation for the Realization of Human Potential.

Stress management for me starts with having self-compassion. I dug into mindfulness and self-compassion through The Mindful Self-Compassion course taught by Drs. Kristen Neff and Chris Germer. They focus on being present by engaging our senses in moment-to-moment experiences, being kind to ourselves, and recognizing our common humanity during difficulties. I've also found journaling to be a therapeutic release and an empowering tool for problem-solving. As we write, we can process and choose our thoughts, which can be a form of self-coaching. Stress management also includes creating downtime to relax. I love being in nature and exercising outdoors. When hiking or 'forest bathing,' I use my senses to be mindful, which creates a sense of peace and well-being while exercising. I've formed outdoor adventure groups in various cities I have lived in, and this has been a great way to build social connections while doing activities I love.

Sharing Lifestyle Medicine With Others and Its Impact on Their Health

I started sharing my new-found knowledge and personal successes with my family first. Around that time, I moved in with my father and hoped that sharing LM principles with him would improve his life as it had mine. My mom used to pour her love into preparing delicious homemade dishes accompanied by fresh salads for our family. Therefore, my father's diet had been mainly whole or unprocessed already. Observing my new food choices began to influence him further. He started increasing his fruit and vegetable servings—especially through smoothies. My dad has always loved making smoothies and especially enjoys my breakfast-in-a-smoothie with fruits, greens, nuts, seeds, cooked oatmeal, and quinoa. We started sharing our smoothies with my aunts, and soon, they were in popular demand by other relatives. For the first time together, my dad and I were intentional and invested in improving our health through diet.

Did you know this about diet and lifestyle?

- A study showed patients with severe heart disease who switched to a whole food diet, eliminated oil, meat products, and dairy (except skim milk and nonfat yogurt), and increased fruits, vegetables, whole grains, beans, and legumes resulted in no heart events over 12 years of observation [8].
- A trial of a 10% fat, whole food vegetarian diet, aerobic exercise, stress management, quitting smoking, and group support led to a reduction in coronary artery narrowing from cholesterol deposits and a decrease in cholesterol [9].

Despite how advanced the West has become in increasing lifespan through medicines and technology, ironically, the diet for longevity includes foods from a "poor man's diet" of beans and lentils! I began preparing meals for us filled with vegetables, legumes, lentils, and fish, without meat, cheese, or added sugars. I hoped my father's heart health would improve with all his dietary changes. I dared to hope for some reversibility of the disease in his coronary arteries, just as studies had shown was possible. Within the first year of his diet change, we felt overjoyed that my father's LDL cholesterol dropped 30 points into the 60s, which was within the ideal range. We were also astounded that his exercise stress test became normal for the first time in years. How validating to witness this reversibility of my dad's heart disease by diet changes alone!

Cooking and eating healthy meals together are wonderful ways to bond with my creative nieces and nephews. Of course, kids gravitate to desserts. I'm delighted whenever my 10-year-old niece, Haleema, shows me her search results for dessert recipes without added sugars that we can bake together. The kids know about my push toward natural sugar. At age four, my niece Ahsiyah would proudly show me when she was eating whole fruits, saying, "See, this is healthy," raising her hand that held a strawberry or apple. One of our favorite activities has been a day trip for strawberry picking, and on the ride back, my niece shared her preference to consume her strawberry pickings in a smoothie, not in a cake. We have since captured that memory in a colorful farm painting, painted together with various size strawberries, now hung up in my home. I feel refreshing joy when I hear the kids choose whole food and nutritious options, realizing they are using information they are learning to make wise food choices.

Even how I host gatherings has been transformed. It's not about keeping up with the Joneses but paving a path toward wellness. Gone are the days of catering or buying store-bought frozen appetizers and packaged desserts. Knowing what I know, I feel responsible for feeding others healthy foods. It takes extra time, but I now prepare food from scratch. My appetizer can start with a fruit salad, and I use dates as the natural sweetener in desserts. For holiday feasts, my primary entrée is vegetable biryani, an Indian delicacy, using my mother's prized recipe—one I've modified by minimizing oil and substituting brown basmati rice instead of white rice. I hope guests realize that eating healthy can still taste good. Acts of service, like cooking, had been my mother's love language. I never imagined that cooking would become my way of treating others to good health, happiness, and, hopefully, longevity.

My desire to share good health habits and surround myself with like-minded people led me to create health-oriented social groups. In my "Mindfully Healthy" group, we post daily to share progress on our goals, including the common group goals of consuming five fruit and vegetable servings and doing moderate-intensity exercise. I created this group to help inspire, support, and celebrate my friends on their health journeys, yet it has been a central touchstone to keep me on track over the years.

I also created a Ramadan Healthy Home Cooked Meal Challenge group to motivate those fasting for the month to stay healthy and active. Ramadan is a month to be mindful of being our best selves. Abstaining from food during the daytime lends itself to spirituality, but feasting at night does the opposite. Eating in moderation is one of the Islamic traditions, to fill the stomach one-third with food and one-third with drink, leaving the last third for air. My Ramadan challenge includes five fruit and vegetable servings, five minutes of moderate-intensity exercise, and 48 ounces of water intake daily. These physical choices keep us light and alert even at the end of a day of fasting. The challenge has been going strong for three years, empowering participants to create and maintain healthy habits.

My allergy and asthma patients often bring up all aspects of their health, including their blood pressure, diabetes, excess weight, and depression, during office visits. We then discuss lifestyle choices that can help these conditions. Asthmatic patients' breathing and lung function can be affected by obesity, or belly fat, which is also referred to as abdominal obesity. When a patient mentions their weight, is obese, or their breathing test shows abdominal obesity has restricted their lung expansion, the conversation then turns toward lifestyle choices affecting their weight. We discuss any relevant diet, exercise, sleep, and emotional health changes that can help.

One patient stands out as someone who changed her health by changing her lifestyle. She had a flare-up of her asthma due to COVID, required prolonged steroids, and went into depression. She started neglecting her health, resulting in weight gain, inactivity, and increased cholesterol. She shared the toll it was taking on her. I made some recommendations, and she changed her diet entirely, started exercising, and got counseling. She joyfully shared her progress and the amazing results a few months later. In a dramatic success story, she improved her mood, lowered her cholesterol, and lost weight, which in turn helped her asthma. She expressed gratitude that my listening to her, being in rapport with her, and discussing the mental and physical aspects of her health helped empower her. In her words, 'It all starts with one small change. Focusing on one thing made all the difference.' She attributes my suggestion to just cut back on her bacon to reduce her cholesterol started the domino effect, after which she also cut back on eggs and more. She shared, 'You never know the impact someone's words can have on the other person to make it click. It opens up a door.'

Some people's health changes are dramatic, and some are gradual. What is important is that the change is sustainable. Simply committing to one action towards a healthy lifestyle and continuing that action over six months is an effective strategy for changing long-term behavior. When one introduces healthy habits into their lifestyle, it crowds out unhealthy ones. Adding a fruit or vegetable into the diet or squeezing in even five minutes of exercise daily is an easy way to start!

Conclusion

Everyone's journey to better health starts somewhere. My parents' medical conditions sparked my interest in lifestyle medicine, which ultimately had a positive ripple effect. I took the reins on my health and turned it around. I invite my friends, family, and readers to do the same. Learning so much about the impact of lifestyle choices on health and disease prevention has been a blessing and an empowering experience.

Knowledge is power. I hope the facts and experiences I've shared inspire and motivate readers toward their health transformations, one action at a time. Join us in the Lifestyle Medicine movement toward personal and global health.

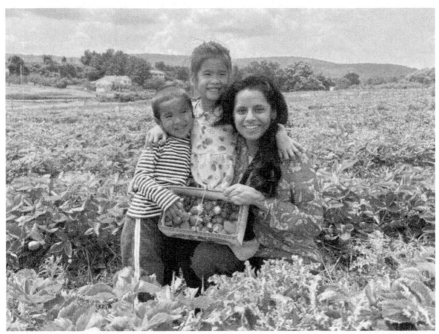

A fun day at the farm picking strawberries with my niece and nephew.

I dedicate this chapter to my parents. My beloved father, Azmat Sharif, has been a pillar of wisdom and sacrifice for my family. My mother, Dr. Rizwana Sharif, my biggest champion, was an example of strength and positivity. They both taught me the value of hard work, excellence, faith, and service.

I also extend deep gratitude to my sister Sana, who, in her kindness and generosity, provided thoughtful input on this story.

References:

1. Benjamin, M. M., & Roberts, W. C. (2013). Facts and Principles Learned at the 39th Annual Williamsburg Conference on Heart Disease. *Baylor University Medical Center Proceedings, 26*(2), 124–136. https://doi.org/10.1080/08998280.2013.11928935.

2. Roberts, W. C. (1995). Preventing and arresting coronary atherosclerosis. *American Heart Journal, 130*(3), 580–600. https://doi.org/10.1016/0002-8703(95)90369-0.

3. Campbell, T. C., Parpia, B., & Chen, J. (1998). Diet, lifestyle, and the etiology of coronary artery disease: the Cornell China Study. *American Journal of Cardiology*, *82*(10), 18–21. https://doi.org/10.1016/s0002 -9149(98)00718-8.

4. Van Der Ploeg, H. P., Chey, T., Korda, R. J., Banks, E., & Bauman, A. (2012). Sitting Time and All-Cause Mortality Risk in 222 497 Australian Adults. *Archives of Internal Medicine*, *172*(6), 494. https://doi. org/10.1001/archinternmed.2011.2174.

5. Eijsvogels, T. M. H., Molossi, S., Lee, D., Emery, M. S., & Thompson, P. M. (2016). Exercise at the Extremes. *Journal of the American College of Cardiology*, *67*(3), 316–329. https://doi.org/10.1016/j.jacc.2015.11 .034.

6. Woodcock, J., Franco, O. H., Orsini, N., & Roberts, I. (2011). Non-vigorous physical activity and all-cause mortality: systematic review and meta-analysis of cohort studies. *International Journal of Epidemiology*, *40*(1), 121–138. https://doi.org/10.1093/ije/dyq104.

7. *2008 Physical Activity Guidelines for Americans | health.gov* . https://health.gov/our-work/nutrition-physical-activity/physical-acti vity-guidelines/previous-guidelines/2008-physical-activity-guidelines.

8. Esselstyn, C. B. (1999). Updating a 12-year experience with arrest and reversal therapy for coronary heart disease (an overdue requiem for palliative cardiology). *American Journal of Cardiology*, *84*(3), 339–341. https://doi.org/10.1016/s0002-9149(99)00290-8.

9. Ornish, D., Brown, S. S., Billings, J. H., Scherwitz, L., Armstrong, W. T., Ports, T. A., McLanahan, S., Kirkeeide, R. L., Gould, K. L., & Brand, R. A. (1990). Can lifestyle changes reverse coronary heart disease? *The Lancet*, *336*(8708), 129–133. https://doi.org/10.1016/0140-6736(90) 91656-u.

About Dr. Saba Sharif, MD, FAAAI, DipABLM

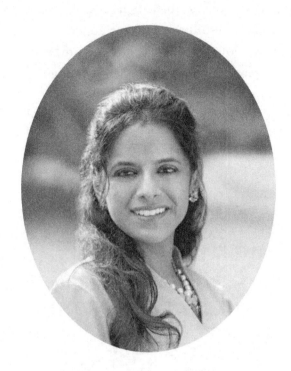

Dr. Saba Sharif completed an accelerated medical program at the Sophie Davis School of Biomedical Education with her clinical years at SUNY Stony Brook School of Medicine, followed by a residency in Internal Medicine at Winthrop University Hospital, all in New York. She then completed fellowship training in Allergy & Immunology from Kaiser Permanente in Los Angeles, CA.

Dr. Sharif has been practicing medicine for over 20 years. She is board certified in both Allergy & Immunology and Lifestyle Medicine. She has earned a Fellow status in the American Academy of Allergy Asthma and Immunology, or FAAAI. The Fellow status is a recognition of achievement and proficiency in the field. As an Allergy, Asthma, and Immunology Specialist, she gets fulfillment from making early diagnosis and treatment decisions and improving patients' quality of life. She enjoys teaching her patients, including any relevant pearls from Lifestyle Medicine.

She is a lifelong learner and believes in a growth mindset. She enjoys experimenting with cooking, challenging herself to create tasty recipes with natural sugar and minimal fat. She adheres to a predominantly pescatarian diet. She loves spending time in nature by hiking and biking. She hopes to inspire and impact others by sharing the transformative lessons of Lifestyle Medicine.

LinkedIn: www.linkedin.com/in/Saba-S-IM-AI-LM

Watch an interview with the co-author:

Co-Author spotlight
DR. SABA SHARIF

Scan Me

29

Self-Care for Better Patient Care: My Journey to Wellness

Mamatha Sirivol, MD, MPH, DipABLM, DipABOM

"Education is the most powerful weapon which you can use to change the world."

— Nelson Mandela

As a young adult, I pursued medicine with the noble thought of treating disease and saving lives. After successfully graduating from medical school with a degree of M.B.B.S, and before starting my residency, I chose to pursue a master's in public health. This avenue luckily gave me an insight into the preventive aspects of disease, more from the public health perspective.

Thereafter, my three-year Family Medicine residency opened up a world of opportunities to learn from the most diverse patient population of all ages and genders. While learning and imbibing knowledge on wellness and sick visits, managing acute infections and chronic diseases, and learning the pathophysiology of a disease and its management, I connected the dots with my public health knowledge. Practicing Family

Medicine for the past 10 years has broadened my knowledge and deepened my understanding of the disease process, and the role lifestyle plays in the development and progression of several diseases.

When the COVID-19 pandemic hit, I decided to do an Obesity Medicine fellowship, focused on trying to do something useful with all the extra time we suddenly had on hand as the entire world came to a halt. But as I delved into the specifics of obesity management and learned the intricacies of the why, what, and how of the causes of disease, my interest in Lifestyle Medicine (LM) grew exponentially. Counseling patients about obesity felt incomplete without discussing the other aspects of their lifestyle and prevention. When I stumbled upon the opportunity to pursue board certification in LM as well, little did I realize that it would change my life, personally and professionally! With a background in Public Health, trained to protect and improve the health of communities through education, a career in LM was the next best step to help individual patients achieve good health.

My classical training always included the full food pyramid. Never before in my life have I felt that an exclusively plant-based diet could still be a well-balanced diet. I have been trained to counsel patients to include protein which we implied must come from animals, and to consume dairy for the body's calcium needs. With my knowledge, I can counsel on nonanimal-based sources of nutrition. After attending the nutritional medicine conference by the Physician Committee for Responsible Medicine (PCRM), my knowledge and affinity for plant-based whole foods grew so much that I have started implementing new standards and practices for myself and my patients.

I have discovered several new aisles in the grocery store that were seemingly inconspicuous before! I enjoy shopping for a wide new variety of colorful vegetables which are a treat to your eyes and the tongue. To list a few examples, I have replaced potato chips with kale chips. My children love the crunch with a touch of sesame. Desserts are replaced by fresh fruit. Other delights include the freshness of broccoli, the wholesomeness of vegetable soup, and air-fried tofu tossed into a salad, to name a few.

I have had chronic low back pain for as long as I remember. I was in my early twenties when my back pain hit me hard, limiting my activities. I would not dare to lift anything more than a few pounds, and I dreaded long drives and had to make special requests to have stools in patient rooms replaced with chairs with back support. Each sciatica flare would take away a few productive days out of my life. It did not surprise me when my MRI showed disc desiccation at a lumbar vertebra.

After years of struggling with back pain, one day, I had an awakening. I wanted to take control of my pain, not with medications or limiting my activity, but with regular exercise and lifestyle changes. Though I was a very physically active person all my life, I started doing daily yoga and slowly increased the duration. It was amazing to personally experience the gradual resolution of my pain and improvement in the range of motion in my back. For the first time in years, I could lie down on the ground and get back up again without support from someone. I was able to sit and squat on the ground for my daily prayers without pain. I was able to sit on a stool without back support and have conversations with patients without worrying about being in pain. The stiffness has been replaced by core strength. In fact, simply not being in pain improved the quality of my life tremendously. I have noticed the resolution of my tension headaches with neck and upper back exercises.

When yoga felt a little less intense as I grew stronger, I added dance workouts to make them more aerobic and more significant in intensity. This has helped me lose a few pounds and a few inches around my waist, something that has not happened in years. When you work so hard to burn calories, you tend to think twice before putting those calories into your mouth unless they are a must. I have experienced that personally. I eat healthily when I exercise. I do not get as hungry. I feel happier. I feel accomplished. I carry positive energy with me, which I share with my patients and anyone I encounter. I have changed the way I shop, the way I cook, the way I eat, and the way I counsel my patients.

A key takeaway I worked on was eating mindfully. I have learned to put away my phone when eating. I educate my kids to do the same. We all, as a family, have been working toward mindfulness practices. I make it a point to educate my patients about mindful eating. Looking at what we eat, relishing the taste and appearance of food, and enjoying every bite make eating so much more enjoyable and satiating.

Regular physical activity, mindful eating, and good sleep hygiene have become my way of life. These have helped me stay healthy and stay content. I always have had good social connections, but an in-depth knowledge of lifestyle medicine helped me make meaningful and lasting relationships and helped me focus on what is important to my mental well-being. I have picked up learning piano by taking formal classes and practicing it, which helps me de-stress. My passion for gardening, outdoor walks, the time I spend with my family, arts and crafts I do with my children . . . everything feels more meaningful due to being more mindful!

Working on my personal progress has been reflected in my professional development. Recently, I have been reading the book *UnDo It* by Dr. Dean Ornish, which has been greatly helpful in expanding my knowledge of lifestyle medicine and educating patients about the role lifestyle plays in reversing chronic diseases.

According to WHO, 80% of heart disease, stroke, type 2 diabetes, and 40% of cancer could be prevented with improvements in diet and lifestyle. Practicing LM and educating patients at the grass root level, that is, in their primary care offices, is a valuable resource to maintain good health, prevent hospitalizations, and lower healthcare costs.

I see tens of patients every day, and it is alarming to see how many patients smoke or have a problem drinking, or have some other vice in their life. What makes it more intriguing is that almost all of them know that smoking, excessive alcohol use, drug use, unhealthy diet, etc., are harmful and could have multiple direct and indirect effects on one's health. But due to a lack of proper education and direction, they continue to struggle. With increasing evidence of the relationship between cancer risk and unhealthy lifestyle and the role lifestyle plays in modifying epigenetics, there is a tremendous need to educate patients and gear them toward healthy, quality living. My lifestyle medicine education has helped me identify such patients by asking the right questions, assessing their readiness, and forming a plan individualized to them.

I have been more successful in treating obesity with the acquired knowledge of lifestyle medicine combined with obesity medicine knowledge. I have enjoyed showing the patients how achieving the target calorie goals is much easier with a plant-based diet than with an omnivorous diet. I have utilized the principles and techniques of motivational interviewing, which helped engage patients better and increase their participation and investment in their health to bring the desired result.

As a family physician, I see patients of all ages. The community that benefits most from counseling and guidance for developing and maintaining a healthy lifestyle is the pediatric population. With pediatric obesity being on the rise, my education in lifestyle medicine equipped me with the right tools to identify and address the problem. I take time to educate children on a healthful diet, physical activity, avoiding risky substances, judicious use of screen time, developing good sleep hygiene, and forming meaningful social relationships. This has helped me bond with my patients strongly, visit after visit.

A secondary benefit of actively practicing Obesity Medicine and Lifestyle Medicine has been the improved quality of my patient encounters and increased patient satisfaction. In the limited time doctors have with patients, it does not take long to stress the major tenets of lifestyle medicine. Assessing the patient's readiness to change, applying a few basic concepts of cognitive behavioral therapy (CBT), and setting SMART goals before they leave the office has helped attain lasting results.

Never have I enjoyed "de-prescribing" as much as I do now. After meeting with me periodically over months and having made sustainable lifestyle changes, patients appreciate being on fewer medications for their chronic diseases, such as diabetes and hypertension, than before. I work with my patients, engage in deep and meaningful conversations, identify an area of change, and make a detailed, well-defined plan with them with a promise to meet them in about eight weeks, which I feel is an optimal interval between visits and works the best to keep patients accountable. It's very rewarding to see how patients have succeeded with this simple yet powerful approach.

A healthy lifestyle should promote not just physical health but also mental and emotional well-being. This concept of positive psychology and social connectedness, which I learned as a part of my lifestyle medicine training, has greatly helped me counsel my patients on improving their social well-being and helping individuals thrive. I encourage them to consider going on a whole food plant-based (WFPB) diet, which has been proven to improve mood and help with depressive symptoms almost on par with medications in some patients. I stress the importance of daily exercise, a regular purposeful physical activity, the benefits of which go much beyond weight loss or being in shape. I discuss various mindfulness-based stress reduction strategies with them, such as picking up a hobby, developing problem-solving skills, learning time management techniques, etc., which improve their overall emotional and physical well-being.

Another aspect of lifestyle medicine I thoroughly enjoyed learning is the role sleep plays in one's health. Sleep has been underrated for decades. Growing up, sleep was often projected as a sign of laziness. Many successful people boasted they "burnt the midnight oil." But with education came awareness and knowledge that sleep is crucial for body systems to function. A good night's sleep rejuvenates the body and boosts one's memory. When patients complain of anxiety or depression, they almost always struggle with insomnia. Identifying sleep disorders, educating patients on the importance of good sleep hygiene, and helping them with a "lifestyle prescription" has been rewarding.

As they say, you educate a man, you educate an individual. You educate a woman, you educate a nation. Guess what happens when you educate a woman doctor?! My training in lifestyle medicine just came at the right time, taking stock of where I have already been and looking forward to the future of medicine, making a difference, one patient at a time!

—◆○◆—

This chapter is dedicated to my family and my friends, who have been my biggest source of strength, support, and inspiration. The patients I interact with have taught me valuable lessons which enriched my perspective and provided a constant reminder of the importance of my work. It was a great pleasure being involved in this project.

—◆○◆—

About Dr. Mamatha Sirivol, MD, MPH, DipABLM, DipABOM

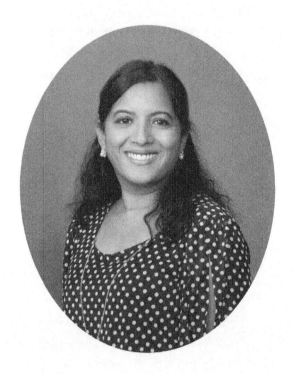

Dr. Mamatha Sirivol is a board-certified Family Physician who currently practices in a hospital-based group practice in the Bangor area in the beautiful state of Maine. Additionally being board certified in both Obesity Medicine and Lifestyle Medicine, she is passionate about practicing and spreading the joy of lifestyle medicine while providing comprehensive medical care for families.

She is married and a proud mother of two beautiful girls and enjoys connecting with people and traveling. When she is not at work, you will find her working out, cooking, gardening, and being proactively involved in community events. She practices self-care with her newfound love of learning piano and is a strong advocate for holistic mindfulness.

Watch an interview with the co-author:

DR. MAMATHA SIRIVOL

Scan Me

30

ADVERSITY, PERMISSION & FINDING PURPOSE

Wendy Stammers (UK), MBCHB, MRCGP, DFSRH, DRCOG, DipIBLM/BSLM

"Always remember you matter, you're important, you are loved and you bring to this world things no one else can."
— The Boy, the Mole, the Fox, and the Horse by Charley Mackesey

"I'm so sorry!" These were the three words that hit my husband and me when my friend broke the bad news in Sheffield Children's Hospital Emergency Department on 23rd December 2019. "Oliver has a brain tumor!" Our youngest son, aged five, had been having intermittent neck pains for the preceding two months and then had the occasional vomit whilst at school. On that fateful day, we were all packed to visit my family in Norfolk for Christmas, and Oliver vomited three times before we left—our suspicions had already been escalating, and we were waiting for a brain scan, but now we couldn't wait. We drove straight to A&E (Accident and Emergency Hospital), and that is where we remained for the following two weeks. Fortunately, we consider ourselves one of the lucky families as Oliver's tumor was benign—a pilocytic astrocytoma. It took several months, but he eventually made a full recovery, and today, he's a healthy, active, and fit eight-year-old boy.

This experience shifted my perspective, and I began to view life through a different lens—one of immense gratitude and purpose. I was filled with a burning desire to seize my life with both hands and as Charley Mackesey would say, "Listen more to my dreams and less to my fears."

Back in December 2017, my dream was ignited when I was traveling in my car and listening to an interview with Dr. Rangan Chatterjee on BBC radio. He was discussing his book, *The Four Pillar Plan*. That interview proved to be a turning point in my career. It was then that I realized where I truly belonged—in the world of Lifestyle Medicine. Dr. Chatterjee's words resonated with me, and the scientific evidence supporting his ideas was strong and compelling. I knew that this was a field that I couldn't ignore.

I immediately ordered the book and started to binge-listen to the *Feel Better Live More* podcast, which he launched in 2018! The show featured interviews with world-renowned specialists like Prof. Satchin Panda, author of *The Circadian Code*, Prof. Tim Spector, author of *The Diet Myth*, *Spoon Fed*, and *Food for Life*, and Prof. Matthew Walker, author of *Why We Sleep*. Each episode was a revelation and filled a crucial gap in my medical toolkit. The ideas and concepts they presented made perfect sense and inspired me to pursue Lifestyle Medicine with even greater passion and dedication.

After Oliver recovered from his brain surgery, I returned to work in August 2020, in the midst of the COVID-19 pandemic. At that time, I had been a General Practitioner (GP) partner for nine years, with two young boys aged eight and five, and a loving and devoted husband. I loved being a GP and helping others, but I had grown increasingly frustrated with the system. I constantly found myself running behind schedule in my 10-minute consultations because I was more interested in helping my patients identify the root causes of their illnesses rather than just treating their symptoms with an ever-increasing number of pharmaceuticals. I firmly believed that many of the patients I saw were suffering from imbalances in their lifestyles and that if they could be equipped with the knowledge and self-belief to address these issues, their symptoms would ease without the need for long-term or lifelong medications. Unfortunately, the constraints of the healthcare system, increasing patient demands, complexities, and lack of resources made it impossible for me to deliver this type of service within our practice.

With newfound permission and determination to pursue my dreams, I realized that I was no longer satisfied with my partnership role, and my ambition to deliver lifestyle medicine to my patients far exceeded the security of general practice. The incredible work of Professor Tim Spector and his colleagues, who gathered COVID-19 pandemic data in the Zoe Health Study, further fueled my hunger for lifestyle medicine. I appreciated the increasing evidence linking disease severity, morbidity, and mortality to lifestyle habits. This made me more determined to advocate for a proactive approach to healthcare and encourage my patients to focus on lifestyle modifications as the foundation of their healthcare journey.

In 2021, I made the bold decision to leave my partnership and pursue my dream of providing lifestyle medicine to my patients. It was at the British Society of Lifestyle Medicine conference in Edinburgh where I found my passion and ambition matched by like-minded individuals who shared my beliefs. This was a pivotal moment in my 20-year career as a doctor, as I finally felt a sense of purpose and belonging. I furthered my expertise by training as a Health and Wellness Coach and eventually became a board-certified lifestyle medicine doctor in December 2022.

With every bit of evidence I was reading and digesting, I recognized the undeniable impact that food and nutrition have on our health and well-being. Hippocrates' famous quote, "Let food be thy medicine and medicine be thy food" suddenly made sense. I, therefore, decided to embark on a journey toward a 90% plant-based diet, not just for my own health but for that of my husband and children too. With the help of Dr.

William Bulsiewicz's *The Fibre Fuelled Cookbook* and Drs. Shireen and Zahra Kassam's invaluable Plant-Based Health Professionals' resources, I discovered the incredible benefits of plants and the magic of herbs and spices. Despite initial resistance from my household, and the added challenge of my husband's long history of an inflamed and sensitive gut, I persisted with determination, honesty, and lots of planning. And guess what? It worked! Our boys are thriving, passionate about maximizing their "plant points," and recognizing the negative impact of processed foods. My eldest son even said to me the other day, "Mummy, I think the school dinners are poisoning us!" My husband's gut health has also markedly improved and he is now able to enjoy lentils, beans, onions, garlic, and other gut-healthy foods without distressing symptoms and discomfort.

What do I mean by plant points, and what is the evidence for this? The American Gut Project analyzed stool samples from over 10,000 citizen scientists worldwide, revealing valuable insights into differences in gut microbes. Notably, those who consumed over 30 types of plant-based foods per week had a more diverse mix of gut microbes than those who consumed fewer than 10. This is significant because greater gut microbe diversity is linked to better health. The term "plant-based" encompasses more than fruits and vegetables; it also includes whole grains, legumes, nuts, seeds, herbs, and spices. While the "5-a-day" guideline for fruit and vegetable intake is a good starting point, it disregards the 40 trillion microbes residing in our gut, which require various plant foods to thrive. Each strain of bacteria performs a different function and favors a specific plant food. Thus, the more diverse plant foods we consume, the more diverse our gut microbes can become, which can enhance our immune system (of which 70% lives in our gut), increase our resistance to infection, fortify our gut barrier, produce vitamins, regulate hormones, communicate with the brain, balance blood sugar, reduce blood fats, and lower the risk of multiple diseases. This is only a glimpse into the vast responsibilities our gut microbes have. It is vital to get in your "plant points!"

The journey wasn't always easy, but the rewards have been immeasurable. Watching my family embrace a healthier way of life and thrive on plant-based meals has filled me with immense pride and inspiration, knowing that they are setting themselves up for a long life of wellness rather than illness.

During this same period, I was fortunate enough to meet Dr. Linda Mizun, a National Health Service (NHS) A&E doctor, and Dr. Adrian Jeyakumar, an NHS GP, both board-certified lifestyle medicine doctors based here in Sheffield, England.

They have become an instrumental part of my journey, and we co-founded **"Hero of Health (HoH),"** a globally scalable, digital platform with the mission to build HoH Healthy Ageing Neighborhoods that fuel sustainable lifestyle changes regardless of one's socioeconomic background. We foster purpose-driven social connections that tackle loneliness, promote mental wellness, and subsequently activate patients to prioritize their health. Once patients become activated, they are ready to engage in our chronic disease reversal programs and activities.

Through our combined 50 years of clinical experience and our very own personal encounters, we've observed that a lack of community purpose breeds loneliness, isolates individuals, and triggers mental health issues. This erodes self-esteem, hampers the desire to make healthy lifestyle choices, and amplifies the risk of chronic illnesses, and thus accelerates aging. Our approach tackles this at its core, emphasizing the vital importance of finding one's purpose. Recognizing humans as inherently social beings, we prioritize enhancing social purpose to foster lasting healthy habits.

Studies have repeatedly shown that people with a sense of purpose in their lives are less likely to develop depression and anxiety and more likely to engage in healthy behaviors such as eating a healthy diet and exercising regularly. Our early clinical findings support our assumption that fostering nurturing neighborhoods facilitates inter-generational social connections that can lead to individuals finding a sense of purpose in life.

This purpose, in turn, empowers them to make the necessary lifestyle changes that address the root cause(s) of their health problems, which in turn brings life back into their years rather than merely adding years to their lives.

Embarking on the task to build a HoH Healthy Ageing Neighbourhood here in Sheffield, UK, we have partnered with Townships One Primary Care Network, a group of forward-thinking GP practices that are passionate about incorporating lifestyle medicine into primary care. Through our partnership, we have established the first HoH Healthy Ageing Neighbourhood, where patients become Heroes by rediscovering their social purpose in their communities. This transformation enables them to reverse chronic diseases, reduce medication reliance, and achieve improved health outcomes for life with the support of their new friends in their neighborhoods.

To unleash the Hero of Health, our app builds social connection locally with 5 simple steps: Online Connection, Walk & Talk, Cooking Together, Chronic Disease Reversal Programs, and the birth of Hero of Health Volunteers. These steps are supported and guided by the Hero of Health Digital algorithms, creating a dynamic and interactive social experience that facilitates the adaptation of sustainable healthy lifestyle habits. We wholeheartedly invite you to join us on our mission to build 1000 Healthy Aging Neighborhoods in the UK by June 2024. By working together, we aim to support health equality, alleviate the pressures on the NHS, and contribute to our overall economic prosperity.

Here are a few stories from the group highlighting how finding purpose, addressing loneliness, and gaining hope impact our mental and physical health (names have been changed to protect their identities):

Mandy, a 65-year-old woman with a complex medical history that includes type 2 diabetes (requiring both tablets and insulin), two heart attacks, a cardiac arrest, obesity, fatty liver disease, depression, and eating disorders, retired on medical grounds and was at a low point after experiencing isolation during the COVID-19 pandemic. Despite being under the care of endocrine specialists for over 10 years, her blood sugar levels remained dangerously high, even with high doses of insulin. Within just 14 weeks of joining the weekly walks, Mandy found a renewed sense of purpose and belonging. As an excellent cook, she began leading and delivering plant-based cooking sessions to the group, benefiting everyone. Her blood sugar levels are now the best they have been in over 15 years, and she is gradually reducing her insulin requirements. Her exercise tolerance has significantly increased, her sleep has improved, and she has even stopped taking her blood pressure medications. Mandy reports that she cannot remember a time when she felt happier.

Brian, a 60-year-old man with a history of anxiety, insomnia, chronic pain, and a recent diagnosis of type 2 diabetes, had to take a break from work due to rising levels of anxiety. After only a few weeks of implementing small yet significant changes to his nutrition and gaining support and connection from the group, Brian's spirit returned, and he started to make progress in improving his health. His wife's health also benefited as she was incredibly supportive and receptive to everything he was learning. He recognized the strong link between lifestyle and mental health, and his anxiety began to reduce. After only a few months, he stopped taking his antidepressants. Brian lost weight, his diabetes is reversing, and he has now returned to work. His fitness has improved considerably, and he can now easily walk 10,000 steps per day, having been inactive for some time. Brian has found a new sense of purpose, he became the lead for the walking groups, enjoying finding new suitable routes, and sharing his lived experience and passion for his newfound health.

Audrey, a 66-year-old lady with type 2 diabetes (requiring tablets and insulin), obesity, chronic pain, and reduced mobility, was reliant on a mobility scooter. She came to us after her husband joined the group the preceding week, and she was impressed by the information shared by him, especially about the effects of processed sugar. He was more concerned about Audrey, who had been consuming 30 teaspoons of sugar per day from adding it to her cups of tea and to her Weetabix in the mornings and before bed. Audrey had developed this sugar addiction during her two-week stay in the hospital after her hip replacement when she was given sugar in her tea, something she had not previously consumed. After joining the program, Audrey attended the group the next week in her mobility scooter and had already stopped consuming sugar in her tea and reduced the amount on her Weetabix to just one tablespoon. She had gone from thirty teaspoons to just six overnight. She was feeling less fatigued and more alert and lost four stones (56 lbs) of weight over four months. Due to the rapid weight loss, she was urgently referred for cancer detection, but nothing was identified. Her significant sugar reduction and improvement in insulin sensitivity were responsible for the weight loss. As a result, her insulin doses have reduced, and she is already having discussions with her practice about stopping insulin, something she previously thought was impossible.

Another impactful story that fueled my desire to make lifestyle medicine more accessible to all patients is that of a close friend, a 43-year-old mother of three beautiful children. She called me in June 2022 with the earth-shattering news that she had Stage 3B ovarian cancer. It had spread to her abdomen, and she faced an uncertain journey of chemotherapy and, depending on her body's response, major surgery. The day she phoned was the day after she had been given her diagnosis, following a CT scan and the results of her biopsy. She was devastated, scared, lost, and not sure where to turn to for advice. I will never forget her pleading words, "Wendy, I just want someone to tell me everything is going to be alright." I knew she had contacted me for my positive, anything is possible, take on life and my knowledge and belief in Lifestyle Medicine. "I want to be a fighter, not a victim." Having let this news sink in, I gathered my thoughts and told her, "No matter what, I am coming on this journey with you, and we are going to find everything we can that will give you the greatest chance in overcoming this." Age was on her side, she was fit and healthy, with no other medical conditions. We were unaware of her genetics, but I shared the concept of epigenetics with her—"your genes load the gun, but it is your lifestyle that pulls the trigger." She was desperate to find out what she could control right here and now. She didn't want to hear any statistics, just what she could be doing. We listened and shared resources between us, and the most impactful for me was the book *Radical Remission* by Dr. Kelly A. Turner—a book of cancer survivors against all odds, and the nine common things they all did in response to being given a terminal diagnosis. *How to Live* by Professor Robert Thomas and the work of Dr. William Li on how to *Eat to Beat Disease* were also incredible resources that helped to bring scientific evidence to support dietary changes that could impact my friend's ability to not only withstand the harsh chemotherapy treatment but also to help assist her body in preventing progression or regrowth of the disease. Now, nine months post-diagnosis, she is doing incredibly well with no visible evidence of disease. We have no idea what the future holds, but I truly believe she is facing this challenge with the best chance, great hope, and positivity based on the empowering knowledge of Lifestyle Medicine in conjunction with conventional medicine.

I truly hope this chapter has given you a real feel for how Lifestyle Medicine has transformed my life, as well as the lives of my loved ones, colleagues, and patients. It took immense courage and determination to pursue my purpose, fueled by the traumatic experience of almost losing Oliver. Identifying and pursuing your purpose in life is essential, and if you're considering Lifestyle Medicine, I encourage you to take the leap. I promise that the impact it will have on your life and the lives of those around you will be truly remarkable, and you will never regret the decision to live your life filled with health and purpose.

In conclusion, Lifestyle Medicine is an inspiring field that recognizes the power of small changes in our daily habits and behaviors to make a big impact on our health, our communities, and our world. By embracing this approach and taking action to improve our own lives, we can create a healthier and more sustainable future for ourselves and generations to come.

—◄◊►—

Dedicated to my wonderful husband Nick, and sons, Jacob and Oliver - through adversity we united, found strength and discovered what truly matters - I will remain forever grateful.

To my family, friends, colleagues and patients - you have supported, encouraged, inspired and taught me to follow my passion and believe in myself - I sincerely thank you for enabling me to find my purpose.

—◄◊►—

References:

Mackesy, C. (2019). *The Boy, The Mole, The Fox and The Horse*. Random House.

Chatterjee, R. (2017d). *The Four Pillar Plan: How to Relax, Eat, Move and Sleep Your Way to a Longer, Healthier Life*. Penguin Life.

Panda, S. (2018). *The Circadian Code: Lose weight, supercharge your energy and sleep well every night*. Random House.

Spector, T. (2015). *The Diet Myth: Why the Secret to Health and Weight

Loss is Already in Your Gut. Abrams.

Spector, T. (2022b). *Spoon-Fed: Why almost everything we've been told about food is wrong.* National Geographic Books.

Spector, T. (2022c). *Food for Life: The New Science of Eating Well, by the #1 bestselling author of SPOON-FED.* Random House.

Walker, M. (2017b). *Why We Sleep: Unlocking the Power of Sleep and Dreams.* Simon and Schuster.

ZOE Health Study. https://health-study.joinzoe.com/.

Bulsiewicz, W., MD. (2022). *The Fiber Fueled Cookbook: Inspiring Plant-Based Recipes to Turbocharge Your Health.* Penguin.

Kassam, S., & Kassam, Z. (2022a). *Eating Plant-Based: Scientific Answers to Your Nutrition Questions Eating Plant-Based.* Hammersmith Books Limited.

Turner, K. A., PhD. (2014). *Radical Remission: Surviving Cancer Against All Odds.* Harper Collins.

Thomas, P. R. (2020). *How to Live: The groundbreaking lifestyle guide to keep you healthy, fit and free of illness.* Hachette UK.

Li, W. W. (2019). *Eat to Beat Disease: The New Science of How Your Body Can Heal Itself.* Hachette UK.

About Dr. Wendy Stammers (UK) MBCHB, MRCGP, DFSRH, DRCOG, DIBLM

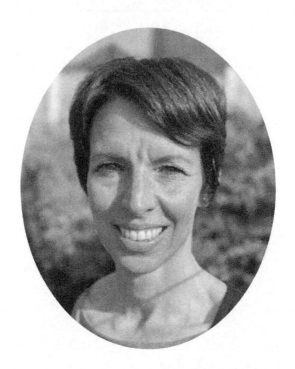

Dr. Wendy Stammers is an NHS GP, Co-Founder of Hero of Health, Board Certified Lifestyle Medicine Doctor, Certified Health and Well-being Coach, mother of two gorgeous, very active boys, and a former GB Age Group Triathlete. She is actively changing the way she practices medicine, empowering patients to find purpose and using evidence-based Lifestyle Medicine to prevent, manage, and reverse chronic diseases.

Website: www.heroofhealth.com/

LinkedIn: www.linkedin.com/in/dr-wendy-stammers/

Instagram: www.instagram.com/hero_of_health

Twitter: www.twitter.com/heroofhealth

Facebook: www.facebook.com/heroofhealthpage

Youtube: www.youtube.com/@HeroofHealth

Watch an interview with the co-author:

Co-Author spotlight
DR. WENDY STAMMERS

Scan Me

31

FINDING BEAUTY IN AN IMPERFECT LIFE

Nandini Sunkireddy, MD, DipABLM, DipABOM

"A fit body, a calm mind, a house full of love. These things cannot be bought – they must be earned."

— Naval Ravikant

Nothing prepares you for having your new baby become a lifelong patient, not even being a doctor. Working as a family physician, I managed to care for my patients and my family. However, when my younger son was born with a severe medical condition, juggling life's many facets was more tenuous than before. He was born with a rare disorder called biliary atresia. This condition ultimately led him to need a liver transplant when he was only six months old. As anyone who has undergone a transplant or had a family member experience a transplant knows, it is not an easy medical procedure. Imagine going through this much medical stress with your young child with a significant medical condition, major medical surgery, and then a post-transplant life full of immunosuppressants to help his little body not reject his transplant. He needed me, but I had to keep working part-time at an urgent care facility. He had many infections, many more surgeries after his transplant, and significant developmental delays, which needed therapy. We were thankful for the occupational and physical therapists who helped him with his flexibility and adjusting to normal infant and toddler developmental milestones like eating and walking.

When he turned three years old, I was able to return to working full-time as a primary care physician, my passion. Many patients were turning to me for help with diabetes and weight loss as these are exploding epidemics in America. I stayed positive and educated them to the best of my ability, but I needed more tools. With the COVID-19 pandemic, even more stress descended on our lives when my father died in September 2020. He passed after battling diabetes and secondary kidney disease for many years and, ultimately, stroke and cardiac arrest. It was overwhelming to watch him struggle with increasing medication doses over the years and progressively become homebound with 12–15 hours of daily peritoneal dialysis and depression. His passing away caused me to re-evaluate my goals for patient care. It became an internal mantra and a tribute to my Dad to try to help patients not endure the same chronic diseases without hope as he suffered. I wish someone had focused on lifestyle changes for his treatment and given him hope that it was possible to treat and reverse diabetes through lifestyle changes.

When I discovered the fields of Lifestyle Medicine (LM) and Obesity Medicine (OM), I knew I had to get certified to help my patients as much as possible. I completed both of these board exams within six months with intense studying. These fields provided tools for me to properly educate and begin coaching my patients on achieving success with their goals for diabetes management and weight loss. My mindset shifted from a knee-jerk reaction of prescribing medications or increasing doses to a long discussion about the six pillars of health through LM. I educated patients about reducing or even eliminating their medications through lifestyle changes. Their eyes lit up at the thought of removing medicines since, previously, they had been sold the idea that they would be on medications for as long as they lived. One such patient was a gentleman who moved from New Jersey to Georgia and was being treated for diabetes and high cholesterol, and he was on six medications, including insulin. After discussing LM, he met with our dietician, who helped with his diet; our exercise physiologist, who got him exercising again; and our psychologist, who helped him stop using food as a coping mechanism for stress. Over a year and with team effort, he lost 20% of his body weight, reduced his medicines to only one blood pressure medication at the lowest dose, was off the insulin, and maintained a healthy lifestyle.

Despite this being my life's passion, my growing practice was taking its toll on me. I was burning the candle at both ends, in my medical practice and at home with my two children, one with special needs and post-transplant medications and doctor's appointments, and all the chores of a typical home. My office in-basket occupied my evenings and weekends, and my husband handled most of the medical appointments for my son. Then, it dawned on me that we were not managing our stress well. Of the six pillars of health that we learned about in LM, we had been vegetarian, physically active, avoided smoking and drinking, slept somewhat reasonable hours, and had a small social circle, but our stress management was not where we needed it to be. At home and work, I felt like a failure, judged based on my "productivity," not my patient outreach and prevention. The hospital quality metrics cannot measure my true impact and its ripple effects throughout the local and now global communities I serve. These "metrics" limited my time off as I could not put myself first. I was not used to saying "no" except to myself and my health needs. I even worked up to a few hours before I went into labor to have my children.

At the near breaking point, I decided to decrease my hours to 0.9 FTE and work four days a week. Now, both my husband and I prioritize 7–9 hours of sleep. I try to be present and experience the moment with more mindfulness. Another daily habit is eating a salad once a day. My husband gave up meat. While I was already vegetarian, I switched to plant-based milk, which has helped my health. We also eat more plant-predominant and whole foods (less processed food). I practice stress reduction techniques like taking long walks and deep breathing.

There was a point when I was so depressed with my son's health that I lost interest in socializing, even though I am an extrovert. Now I realize the importance of social connections on our mental health. So I meet my friends more often, and I love to share LM and have even helped several friends become board certified in LM. My advice for people struggling to make lifestyle changes is to take one day at a time and celebrate small wins. Of course, you need to have a long-term goal in mind, but taking one day at a time and making small changes helps you achieve your long-term goal.

When I put myself and my family first, I could share my message more broadly, maximizing my ability to help patients and grow my practice. With that little time I have "off," I started my YouTube channel, *Style Your Health MD*, to help my patient and community outreach to spread messages of prevention in my native language and English. I can reach many more people with each speaking opportunity and improve the public's health through education, the most powerful tool we have as physicians to impact change in our patients, friends, and family. As many studies have shown about employee productivity, my productivity also increased with less work, although I was still working four days a week. Stress management is a crucial pillar to help achieve the optimal health we all need. We must prioritize our well-being and our family before anything else. The future of medicine is already shifting toward a wellness model rather than a sickness model. Treating and preventing the root cause of disease with lifestyle changes is the key. I wish we had known more about Lifestyle Medicine 30 years ago; my dad would have been with us today and would have enjoyed his golden years of retirement. I hope my story inspires you to keep learning, growing, and caring for yourself and your loved ones by utilizing the six pillars of LM.

*My chapter is dedicated to my son
Anirudh, who is a miracle child, and
in spite of all his surgeries, he always
has a smile on his face.*

About Dr. Nandini Sunkireddy, MD, DipABLM, DipABOM

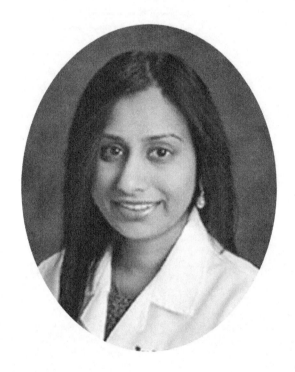

Dr. Nandini Sunkireddy is a Family Physician, board certified in Obesity Medicine and Lifestyle Medicine, the founder of the *Style Your Health MD* YouTube channel, and a paid speaker. I am passionate about introducing patients to the fields of LM and OM and helping them take control of their lives. I love speaking on stage and sharing my message with people who are not my patients. I live in Georgia with my husband and two children. Contact me at <u>styleyourhealthmd@gmail.com</u> to come to speak at your event or to your community.

Website: <u>https://styleyourhealthmd.com</u>

YouTube: <u>https://youtube.com/@styleyourhealthmd</u>

Watch an interview with the co-author:

DR. NANDINI SUNKIREDDY

Scan Me

32

THE SKIN HEALTH SOLUTION, HEALING FROM WITHIN

Yolandas Renee Thomason, DO, DipABLM, DipABOM

"Authenticity is a collection of choices that we have to make every day. It's about the choice to show up and be real. The choice to be honest. The choice to let our true selves be seen."

— Brené Brown

I'm Dr. Renee Thomason, and I'm on a mission to empower women with chronic skin conditions to take charge of their health and become more secure and confident about showing their true selves. I've experienced both sides of the skin health equation. As a doctor, I'm highly trained in understanding the health of the skin from a scientific perspective. At the same time, I'm also a proud skin warrior—I've dealt with a skin condition known as alopecia areata since I was a child. Being diagnosed with alopecia as a youth was hard. I describe my journey with alopecia as an "emotional roller coaster" full of ups and downs because I never knew if I would wake up with a new patch of hair loss or when my hair would grow back. When my hair started falling out, the only thing

I wanted to do was hide it. All the way through my teen years and into young adulthood, I wore wigs every day in order to cover up my hair loss. I was constantly terrified that people would learn the truth about my condition and that they'd reject me because of it. I couldn't even stand to look at myself in a mirror without a wig on.

The shame about my body led me into a downward spiral. I started overeating as an emotional comfort technique. I went up and down in my weight (yo-yo dieting)—I'd crash diet and lose some of the extra weight, then binge eat and gain it all back. My health slowly deteriorated. I developed prediabetes and high cholesterol due to destructive habits and underlying inflammation, even though I was only in my 20s. I even started having stomach problems. As a doctor, I've seen how common this type of situation is when people feel shame about their bodies. The anxiety leads them to respond in unhealthy ways, which makes their health situation even worse, especially if they are living with a chronic skin condition. Maybe you've experienced this yourself. It's easy to feel trapped in a cycle and to feel as if there is no way out. That's how I felt in my early 20s, but then something happened that changed my life. My son was born. I looked at myself through his eyes, and I knew that this wasn't the type of life I wanted him to experience. I wanted to see him become vibrant and confident, ready to show the world his true authentic self, but that wasn't the example I was setting at all. I was trapped in shame and slowly killing myself through bad habits, chronic inflammation, and a poor mindset.

I knew that I needed to make a change in my life after realizing that I wanted to be the best version of myself for my son. This led me to dive deep into research about health and wellness, with a particular focus on skin health and autoimmunity. As I learned more, I began to make positive changes in my life. I decided to pursue a certification in Obesity Medicine, which taught me about the complex pathophysiology of obesity and how mental health plays a significant role in physical health. I applied this knowledge to my own goals and successfully lost a significant amount of weight, both physically and mentally. As a result, my cardiometabolic profile also improved, and I am no longer prediabetic. I then transitioned my career to work as an Obesity Specialist at the Bariatric Clinic in my local hospital, where I find joy in helping others reach their goals. However, I noticed that my patients, and even myself, initially experienced significant weight loss, but it wasn't sustainable since they lacked the daily tools needed for lifestyle modifications.

After achieving significant weight loss and improvements in my labs, I realized that I needed to take a step back and consider the bigger picture of my long-term health goals. I understood that depression and cardiometabolic disease required more than just medication and temporary solutions. It was then that a mentor introduced me to the American College of Lifestyle Medicine (ACLM), where I learned about the six pillars of building a healthy lifestyle. I embraced the pillars of nutrition, exercise, stress management, avoiding risky behavior, getting restorative sleep, and establishing meaningful relationships. Implementing these principles into my life brought a significant improvement in my overall well-being and skin health. As a physician, I knew that these same principles could help my patients achieve similar results, and I began to integrate them into my practice, empowering others to take charge of their health and skin conditions.

Embracing the principles of Lifestyle Medicine (LM) has truly transformed my life. Through focusing on nutrition, I have learned to make healthier food choices that nourish my body and support my overall well-being. Regular exercise has not only helped me maintain a healthy weight but also improved my mental health and mood. Managing stress has become a priority, and I have developed various tools and techniques that help me cope with everyday challenges. Avoiding risky behaviors such as smoking and excessive alcohol consumption has also played a significant role in improving my health. Adequate restorative sleep has become a nonnegotiable aspect of my daily routine, and I prioritize it to ensure that I am functioning at my best. Finally, establishing meaningful relationships and connections with loved ones has brought me immeasurable joy and fulfillment. These LM principles have not only benefited me personally but also helped me become a better physician, as I am now able to guide my patients toward making similar positive changes in their own lives.

As I continued to incorporate LM principles into my own life, I became increasingly aware of the connection between the mind, gut, and skin. I noticed that my own skin health improved as I made changes to my nutrition, sleep, and stress management. This sparked my interest in helping others who were struggling with chronic skin conditions. I realized that many patients were frustrated with the traditional medical approach, which typically involves prescribing medications that may only provide temporary relief. With this in mind, I decided to create the *Mind Gut Skin Academy*, a program that focuses on the connection between lifestyle and skin health. Our goal is to empower individuals living with chronic skin conditions by providing them with the tools and support they need to make sustainable lifestyle changes. Through our program, we aim to help our clients achieve better gut health, reduce inflammation, and ultimately improve their skin health and overall well-being.

I feel incredibly grateful for the opportunity to share my passion for LM with my patients. Many of them come to me with a complex medical history, including trauma, abuse, mental health concerns, and obesity-related complications. Despite these challenges, they all share a common goal: to improve their health and well-being. One patient, in particular, stands out in my mind, a Class 3 obesity patient with uncontrolled depression and a long list of obesity-related medications. Through an individualized 12-week program focused on the pillars of Lifestyle Medicine, we were able to address her mental fitness and emotional eating habits while also providing tools to help her overcome these challenges. Witnessing her transformation has been one of the greatest joys of my career. I have many similar stories of patients who have seen significant improvement in their overall health, particularly those battling chronic inflammatory skin conditions. It was this experience that led me to create the *Mind Gut Skin Academy,* where we focus on the three pillars of skin health: mindset, gut health and nutrition, and lifestyle. My hope is that through sharing my story and the resources I have created, I can inspire others to take a holistic approach to their health and well-being and realize that they, too, have the power to make sustainable changes in their lives.

In conclusion, my journey toward adopting a Lifestyle Medicine approach to health has taught me several valuable lessons. First and foremost, taking a holistic approach to health is crucial for achieving long-term, sustainable changes. By focusing on nutrition, exercise, stress management, avoiding risky behaviors, restorative sleep, and meaningful relationships, I have been able to improve not just my physical health but also my mental and emotional well-being. Through my personal experiences, I have been inspired to create the *Mind Gut Skin Academy*, which is dedicated to educating others on the connection between the mind, gut, and skin and how LM can improve overall health and well-being. I believe that by empowering individuals with knowledge and tools to make positive changes in their lives, we can create a ripple effect that extends beyond just personal health but also positively impacts the community and the world at large. For readers interested in learning more about LM and the *Mind Gut Skin Academy*, I recommend checking out resources such as the American College of Lifestyle Medicine and the *Mind Gut Skin Academy* website. By adopting a Lifestyle Medicine approach to health, I hope to inspire others to prioritize their health and well-being and make positive changes in their lives that lead to long-term, sustainable improvements in health and overall quality of life.

I want to dedicate my chapter to my Grandmother. Thank you for loving me and showing me How to walk with God. I love you always and forever.

About Dr. Yolandas Renee Thomason, DO, DipABLM, Di-pABOM

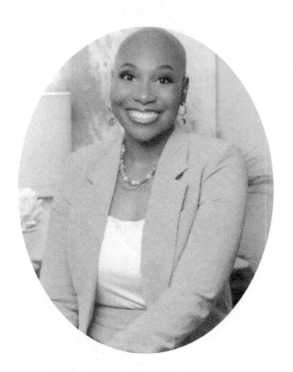

Dr. Renee Thomason is a triple board-certified physician, owner of the *Mind Gut Skin Academy*, and a passionate advocate for women with chronic skin conditions. Diagnosed with alopecia areata at a young age, she understands the emotional and physical toll that chronic skin conditions can have. Dr. Thomason's personal experience inspired her to become the first graduate in her family, complete her MSc, and pursue medical school. Her expertise in Family Medicine, Obesity, and Lifestyle Medicine allows her to help patients improve their gut health and lifestyle, ultimately leading to a better quality of life. Her ultimate goal is to empower women to take charge of their health, feel confident in their skin, and build a supportive community. Dr. Renee is dedicated to using her knowledge and experience to help others heal and live their best lives.

Website: https://www.mindgutskin.com/

Facebook: https://www.facebook.com/drreneethomason

Instagram: https://www.instagram.com/drreneethomason/

LinkedIn: https://www.linkedin.com/in/dr-renee-thomason-7958a22
17/

Watch an interview with the co-author:

Co-Author spotlight
DR. RENEE THOMASON

Scan Me

33

EXTENDING YOUTH: PATHWAYS TO A LONGER, HEALTHIER LIFE

Jaya Venkataraman, MD, FAAP, DipABLM

"We can live a shorter life with more years of disability, or we can live the longest possible life with the fewest bad years."
— Blue Zones Author Dan Buettner

"I t just takes willpower." That was what I constantly was told, told myself, and was trained to tell my patients. I have struggled with body image issues, being overweight, and trying every medically safe way to be healthier and thinner.

I was born a whopping nine and a half pounds—almost unheard of for a baby born to middle-class parents in India. I went on to become a chubby baby all the way to a slightly plump teenager. When I was 13, I was more self-conscious and totally changed my habits and diet and got to a more "normal" weight. My childhood was spent in Africa and Jamaica, where our way of life was to spend countless hours outdoors exploring the great outdoors, exploring nature, and searching for new and interesting bugs, playing cricket with a bamboo stick and tennis ball until we were called to come inside when it was getting dark. At the end of the day, we were so exhausted, and staying up late would have been an impossibility, leaving almost no opportunity for varied sleep schedules.

Weekends and many evenings were spent gardening together as a family. We grew a lot of "Indian vegetables," such as viper snake gourd, valor beans, and greens that were hard to come by. Snacks usually consisted of raw or ripe (depending on the season) mango or unusual fruits such as rose apples, Barbados cherries, sweetsop, breadfruit, soursop, and jack-fruit. Meals were vegetable-intensive and abundant in lentils, herbs, and complex carbohydrates. Treats were often healthy and always in small portions. Drinking water was a natural way to quench the thirst from spending hours in the outside sun.

I grew up vegetarian in environments where fresh vegetables and fruit were abundant, both in the marketplace and in our expansive vegetable garden and the many fruit trees in our backyard and around our home. Interestingly, **all** the food we ate was organic because chemical farming had not yet reached Africa and Jamaica. Growing the food we ate was good exercise and was a part of daily living. Playing outdoors—cricket, tag, badminton, etc.—was a daily activity we looked forward to and not planned "exercise time." Little did I realize then that this was a "blue zones" way of living and what our bodies need.

I went on my first "diet" in my mid-teens and became underweight and too thin. This was the first time I used food as a form of control in my life—something I had to work hard at shaking off as I learned Lifestyle Medicine principles. My exposure to Lifestyle Medicine (LM) came, surprisingly, from one of my interns. LM offers a variety of ways to make better choices. As someone who loves learning, I was eager to learn more. LM gave me tools to help myself and my patients make better choices, and it was liberating to know that it wasn't just about willpower.

The stress of medical school caused me to skip meals frequently, which led to a dangerously low body mass index (BMI). After completing medical school, I immigrated to the United States and experienced the typical immigrant lifestyle of eating more junk food and exercising less. I stayed skinny into my mid-twenties when I gained weight again and kept adding on pounds every decade. As a physician who has counseled children on healthy habits, I was deeply disappointed that I could not be the best role model for the children in my practice and their parents. I also, unfortunately, went through a prior abusive marriage, which started me on a cycle of stress-induced unhealthy eating that I still struggle with, even though it has been over 30 years. Again, this teaches me that traumatic experiences can be a work in progress to heal.

I suffered from decades-long insomnia that only got worse each year. Melatonin supplements were not effective, and as a physician, I did not want to go down the path of daily medication for sleep since they are really only for occasional or short-term use. But in just six months of lifestyle changes, which included getting out for an early evening walk with my now husband, my sleep started to improve. Conversations flow so easily, and the benefits are numerous, from improved relationships to less time spent watching TV after dinner. The soaking up of the sun helps the skin make vitamin D, and the combination of sun exposure and exercise helps with the onset of sleep. Going for a walk after dinner is also supposed to help ward off diabetes, and this seems to have worked so far!

Simply adding this, I was able to overcome my chronic insomnia and start sleeping better. This led to measurable improvements in my blood pressure, cholesterol, and A1C levels. These results motivated me to become a board-certified LM doctor and offer comprehensive pathways to health for my patients, utilizing the six pillars of health.

One of my early patients in my LM practice was a woman in her 50s who had gained about 50 pounds in the last two decades and felt trapped in a vicious cycle of yo-yo diets. She had all but given up when she came to see me and was prepared for a life of medications to deal with diabetes and heart disease. She struggled with feeling like a failure because she could not sustain the willpower to stay on course to lose weight. My counseling, using LM, gave her tools that finally worked—being more mindful about sleep habits, focusing on everything she needs to eat and ideas for practical food prep, small, steady, sustainable steps toward increasing physical activity, and setting SMART goals. She has lost 15 lbs and is steadily continuing to make improvements in her health numbers with lifestyle changes. She still "falls off the plan" but is able to get back on track and no longer spirals.

When I read *The Blue Zones Solution* by Dan Buettner, I realized that my childhood way of living was something I longed for now and needed to extend into my adult life and retirement. I want to play more, garden more, and wander for fun over watching TV or other more sedentary activities. As I read the book, I realized that I just have to step back to my childhood to understand what is needed for a more fulfilling life. The book reminded me that it is the little things in life that give me the most happiness, such as watching a bird sing and harvesting fruits and vegetables from my garden. Spending time with my extended family brings me more happiness than fancy vacations.

I have learned to appreciate these simple pleasures, and I believe that they are essential to a happy and fulfilling life. When I am surrounded by nature, I feel at peace and connected to something larger than myself. When I spend time with my loved ones, I feel loved and supported. And when I help others, I feel a sense of purpose and satisfaction.

As a physician, my advice to my patients who struggle to lose weight has changed from the awful "Eat healthier and exercise more" to meaningful conversations about small incremental lifestyle changes that are sustainable over time, leading to success and feeling and being healthier. I see entire families adopting healthier habits and am hopeful that LM can help reverse the concerning recent trend of decreasing life expectancy in the United States.

Heart disease is a major cause of death in older people, but it can start in the teen years. Emphasizing a healthy diet and good lifestyle habits, including exercise early in childhood, can start a lifetime of heart health. As a pediatrician and Lifestyle Medicine Physician, I am passionate about helping my patients set the foundation for a lifetime of healthy living. I believe that the most important thing we can do for our health is to make small changes that add up over time, starting as early as possible. These changes can include eating a healthy diet, exercising regularly, and getting enough sleep, which we need to instill in our youth.

I am grateful for the opportunity to help my patients make these changes. I have found that the most important thing I can do is to be kind and compassionate. I believe that everyone has the right to live a healthy and fulfilling life. I want my patients to feel supported and encouraged on their journey to better health.

As Dan Buettner says, "We can live a shorter life with more years of disability, or we can live the longest possible life with the fewest bad years." By making small changes to our lifestyle, we can choose the latter, and together, we can create a healthier future for ourselves and for our children.

This chapter is dedicated to my parents, Subramanian and Nagalakshmi Venkataraman, my children, and all my other family.

References:

Buettner, D (2015). The Blue Zones Solution: Eating and Living like the world's healthiest people. National Geographic Books.

About Dr. Jaya Venkataraman, MD, FAAP, DipABLM

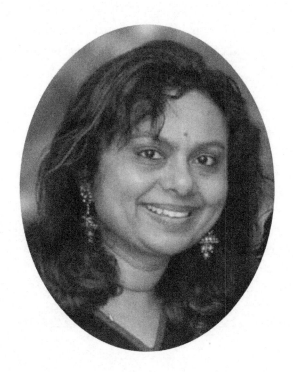

Dr. Jaya Venkataraman is a caring and compassionate board-certified pediatrician at Germantown Pediatric and Family Medicine LLC in Germantown, Tennessee. She has over 20 years of experience in caring for children and young adults.

While she enjoys practicing all areas of pediatrics, she is especially interested in the management of patients with asthma and preventive medicine. Her focus is to help all children develop healthy lifestyle habits so they can live their best lives now and invest in their future health.

Dr. Jaya Venkataraman grew up in India, Tanzania, Jamaica, and Nigeria. Soon after graduating from Obafemi Awolowo University College of Health Sciences in Nigeria, Dr. Venkataraman moved to the United States. She completed her pediatric residency at Henry Ford Hospital in Detroit, Michigan, and worked as an attending physician at the Hospital Clinic for about two years thereafter.

Dr. Venkataraman began practicing in Memphis, Tennessee, at Le Bonheur Children's Hospital in the Pediatric Emergency room and its urgent care centers before starting her practice with a mission to provide excellent personalized care to children. The clinic expanded to take care of patients of all ages recently.

Dr. Venkataraman is a Fellow of the American Academy of Pediatrics and a Diplomate of the American Board of Lifestyle Medicine. She is married with two grown children. Her hobbies include gardening, growing tropical plants, and hiking. Her dream is to visit all 63 US National Parks.

Website: https://www.germantownphysicians.com/provider/jaya-venkataraman-md

LinkedIn: https://www.linkedin.com/in/jaya-venkataraman-bb97a12a

Facebook: https://www.facebook.com/germantownphysicians/

Watch an interview with the co-author:

Co-Author spotlight
DR. JAYA VENKATARAMAN

Scan Me

34

RESOURCES

L earn all about Lifestyle Medicine on the American College of Lifestyle Medicine website and how to become certified whether you're a doctor, nurse, or health coach!

ACLM. (2023b, April 5). *Home | American College of Lifestyle Medicine*. American College of Lifestyle Medicine.

https://www.lifestylemedicine.org/

Nutrition Resources:

Nutrition Facts by Dr. Michael Greger, MD. https://nutritionfacts.org/

Physician Committee for Responsible Medicine by Dr. Neal Barnard: https://www.pcrm.org/

- International Conference on Nutrition in Medicine

- Nutrition for Women's Health Webinar

- 2023 Food for Life Licensing Training Course

- Free CME on their site about nutrition

Plant-Based Nutrition. eCornell.

https://ecornell.cornell.edu/certificates/nutrition/plant-based-nutritio
n/

Ornish Lifestyle Medicine. Ornish Lifestyle Medicine.

https://www.ornish.com/

Physical Activity Resources:

Physical Wellness Toolkit. (2022, December 8). National Institutes of
Health (NIH). https://www.nih.gov/health-information/physical-wel
lness-toolkit

Partnership For A Healthier America. (2023, March 7). *Partnership For
A Healthier America.* Partnership for a Healthier America.

https://www.ahealthieramerica.org/

Stress Management Resources:

3 Tips to Manage Stress. (2022, July 26). www.heart.org
. https://www.heart.org/en/healthy-living/healthy-lifestyle/stress-man
agement/3-tips-to-manage-stress

Manage Stress - MyHealthfinder | health.gov. (2021, August
1). https://health.gov/myhealthfinder/health-conditions/heart-health
/manage-stress

*Tips for Coping with Stress|Publications|Violence Prevention|Injury Cen-
ter|CDC.* https://www.cdc.gov/violenceprevention/about/copingwit
h-stresstips.html

Restorative Sleep Resources:

Good Sleep Habits. (2022, September 13). Centers for Disease Control
and Prevention. https://www.cdc.gov/sleep/about_sleep/sleep_hygien

e.html

Troy, D. (2021, April 2). *Healthy Sleep Habits - Sleep Education by the AASM*. Sleep Education. https://sleepeducation.org/healthy-sleep/he althy-sleep-habits/

Social Connection Resources:

Social Connectedness: National Center for Chronic Disease Prevention and Health Promotion (NCCDPHP)'s Program Successes | CDC. https://www.cdc.gov/chronicdisease/healthequity/sdoh-and-chronic-d isease/nccdphp-and-social-determinants-of-health/social-connectednes s.htm#:~:text=When%20people%20or%20groups%20have,adversity%2 C%20anxiety%2C%20and%20depression

How Right Now. Finding What Helps.

https://www.cdc.gov/howrightnow/

Avoidance of Risky Substances Resources:

How to Quit Smoking. (2023, March 3). Centers for Disease Control and Prevention. https://www.cdc.gov/tobacco/campaign/tips/qu it-smoking/index.html

Home | Smokefree. https://smokefree.gov/

SAMHSA's National Helpline. Substance Abuse and Mental Health Services Administration. https://www.samhsa.gov/find-help/national -helpline

ASAM - American Society of Addiction Medicine.

https://www.asam.org/

Many other references and books are listed in the individual chapters included in this book. Please read all the chapters and references to learn more! Many of the resources listed have local state resources, too, which are not listed here. Please reach out to your state and local sections for more local support.

"Recovery is about progression, not perfection."

— Unknown

Check Out

our
Guide to Wellness Journey
WORKBOOK

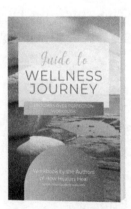

on Amazon

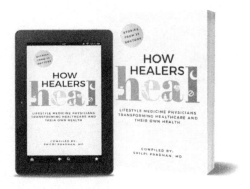

THANK YOU FOR READING THIS BOOK! PLEASE LEAVE A REVIEW!

If you love this book, please share it with a loved one and take your first step toward your future self!

Please leave a 5-star rating on Amazon and write a review on Amazon or wherever you bought this book to help spread inspiration and knowledge! We appreciate it!

Leave a Review!

Scan Me